TESTIMONIALS

"Miriam's voice of experience resonates with all of us who have struggled through a lifetime of dieting. This hands-on approach to keto and low carb eating addresses the hardcore principles, along with providing step-by-step approaches to creating a keto/low carb lifestyle rather than a diet. Helpful meditations and reinforcing affirmations guide one through the hard times. Miriam acknowledges her own life-long struggles with weight loss providing an empathetic underlying tone, as she buoys the reader with encouragement. Breaking Free From Diet Prison: Common Sense Keto and Low Carb is a terrific resource for eliminating the diet roller coaster."

—MARSHA S., FORMER LIFE-LONG DIETER

"Reading the new habits and thoughts made me reflect back on my why and whether I was still honoring it. Had I honestly modified it? Was it still my why and should I be more reflective? Without a why, how do you proceed? It reminded me and gave a fresh perspective in planning meals, not cooking so much that I would tire of leftovers, keeping it simple, and with simplicity, choosing a variety that would keep me moving in the direction of my goals, wishes and dreams. Sometimes practices fall by the wayside and taking ownership of these things resonated with me. I see more success and confidence in my future with more tools at my disposal."

—ELAINE R.

"Each chapter in PART 5 is an element of a toolbox followed by an in-depth explanation, many with detailed worksheets. Beginning in CHAPTER 19: YOUR WHY, all the way to CHAPTER 26: YOUR RELATIONSHIP WITH YOURSELF, I was struck by how wonderfully each element complements the other. "Your Relationship with Yourself" is a crucial part of any health journey. Miriam emphasizes that how we relate to ourselves is even more important than how we relate to food – and once again, gives personal testimony to that fact. I want to emphasize that one of the reasons this book is chock-full of practical, applicable and do-able advice is because it truly illustrates much of Miriam's own health journey to which I can testify because we shared much of the same journey together for more than a decade. She is the quintessential writer, teacher and coach, and for this reason, I value all that she has shared with me in the past and look forward to learning more with her in the future!"

—ELIZABETH S.

"Miriam takes you step-by-step through the process of identifying one's own personal reasons for committing to keto and ultimately how to set and achieve goals. Practical suggestions and worksheets are offered to guide the reader in this process. This is not only a book about keto, but you may learn some things about yourself and some thoughtful life lessons along the way!"

— GAIL S.

"I just wanted to let you know you have done an amazing job. The chapters on meal planning and grocery shopping are very comprehensive and will set readers up for success."

— DANIELLE C.

Breaking Free From Diet Prison

Common Sense Keto and Low Carb

Miriam Hatoum

Gutsy Badger Publishing
Cheyenne, WY

Breaking Free From Diet Prison/Miriam Hatoum

Published by Gutsy Badger Books
gutsy-badger-books.com

ISBN: 978-1-943721-21-4

Photography by Patti Anne Photography
pattiannephotography.com

Book interior and cover design by Ellen Davis
keybookdesign.com

DEDICATION

To my husband, Joe, who has loved me through everything – all the foods, all the diets, all the clothing sizes and all the recipes. Without his love and support I am not sure I could have made it when I did not love myself. …45 years and counting…
Love, Your Dabouli

ACKNOWLEDGEMENTS

Thank you to…

My husband Jawdat who, for more than 40 years, has loved me through every diet I have ever been on. He is my chef and grocery shopper and would never cook anything without first asking, "Can you have this?" He has supported all my endeavors, not the least of which has been Granny Keto, the writing of this book and my new website and course.

My children, Ida and Sami, son-in-law Chris, and especially my grandchildren – the lights of my life – Piper and Owen.

My brothers, Ken and Dan, and especially my sister Susan, who made my current life – living on the beach and running a business – possible.

My sister-in-law Andrea, who was one of my first keto clients. She immediately did everything I suggested and took off running! As a matter of fact, the way she did keto make me realize that you do not have to weigh, measure or track your food in order to lose weight.

My friend Karen from Connecticut (yes, that's her name) for being my very first client when I was getting my coaching certification. Like my sister-in-law Andy, she showed me it is possible to have success without counting, weighing and measuring every morsel – just follow the roadmap!

My girlhood friend, Marsha Shufrin, for also being a client. She had already started her keto journey but had faith in me to carry her further. I can never thank her enough for all the proofreading she did with me for this book.

Lisa Carroll, my keto coach. Her support, patience and knowledge have been immeasurable. Not only is she a great keto coach, but I could not have created my new website and course without her help and encouragement.

Renée Jones, another fabulous coach, who helped me move and remove blocks using forgiveness and insight. I thank her for infusing me with the courage to finish writing this book.

Team Granny Keto: My dear friend, Amy Smith – on so many levels. From setting up my Mac computer and answering hundreds of tech questions so I could get Granny Keto started, to the self-exploration we have done together during our Monday morning book club. Kerry Thompson for her wonderful website design, advice and proofreading. She has been an invaluable go-to person since the day Amy introduced us and we got to work on Granny Keto.

Andrea Hogarth, my dear friend, who has been my legal advisor, friend and supporter throughout the entire process from setting up Granny Keto LLC to publishing this book, to my new website, MiriamHatoum.com with my course, *Breaking Free From Diet Prison: The Roadmap to Low Carb and Keto Success*™.

Amy Berger, who has written the foreword for this book, and who has given me enhanced perspectives on many things. I thank her for her wisdom in taking the crazy out of keto, and her dedication to this lifestyle and her in-depth research (and book) on what is now considered type 3 diabetes: Alzheimer's Disease.

Ellen Davis, my publisher, who has the proverbial "patience of a saint" who was on top of everything, worked closely with me and answered hundreds of questions and worked through dozens of revisions.

Patti Anne Driscoll, my photographer, who captured my essence and inner beauty making me feel as beautiful on the outside.

Dixie Vogel and D.J. Foodie (K.E. William), who were more than generous with their advice about publishing this book.

Jimmy Moore and Daisy Brackenhall, both of whom gave me the courage to find my voice when I first started Granny Keto.

Pioneers in helping us realize that obesity and diabetes are metabolic diseases and not moral issues: Dr. Sarah Hallberg, Dr. Eric Westman, Dr. Dominic D'Agostino, Dr. Robert Atkins, Dr. Jason Fung, Dr. Stephen Phinney, Dr. Jeff Volek and the person responsible for my own lightbulb moment: Gary Taubes. There are so many more people who have been pioneers but these are the few from whom I got my first layer of knowledge, and who prompted me to continue my quest to learn more.

Current pioneers who are helping us understand that the issues at hand are metabolic in nature: Dr. Ken Berry and Dr. Robert Cywes. I thank them both for their insights and for presenting things in easily understandable ways.

Ask Nurse Cindy (Cindy Mikolajczyk) and her daughter Rachael Dee Thomas, for being so generous with the content that they put out.

Kristie Sullivan for being a wonderful and dedicated recipe developer and for being so open and honest with her own journey and for sharing it all so that we can grow and learn and cook!

And finally, Wayne Dyer, Tony Robbins and Mary Morrissey whose books, lectures and seminars showed me ways to harness what I needed to put my knowledge on the printed page.

As I am writing out these acknowledgements, I realize that there are so many more people I could thank for the knowledge and encouragement they have so generously shared. My apologies for not including everyone who has touched my mind and my heart!

TABLE OF CONTENTS

FOREWORD

Low carb and ketogenic diets have exploded in popularity during the past few years. This comes with pros and cons: on the positive side, the avalanche of information available now means that people have instant access to more than they could ever want to know about how these ways of eating work. On the negative side, for every trustworthy and scientifically sound recommendation, there are even more myths, false promises, and advice that is downright dangerous. With so many thousands of blogs, podcasts, books, videos, and other sources putting out information, it's difficult to know whom to turn to for clarity and sensibility. Miriam Hatoum, a.k.a. "Granny Keto," is a welcome voice of reason and reality in a field that daily becomes more alarmist and sensationalist. (Not to mention overwhelming and confusing!)

But where to start? If you're brand new to keto, should you jump right in and completely overhaul your kitchen overnight? What if you want to experience the benefits of lower carb eating but you'd also like to enjoy the fabulous fresh fruit from the local farmers' market in summer, or an occasional serving of black beans and rice at your favorite Mexican restaurant? Can these things co-exist—having improved metabolic health and losing weight without banishing every last molecule of sugar or starch from your diet? Yes, they can! This book will show you how.

Miriam's personal story of transformation will resonate with many of you. A lifetime of yo-yo dieting, calorie counting, and dedicated exercise resulted not in the expected weight loss and better health, but rather, in frustration, disappointment, and self-loathing. Enter the low carb way of eating, and Miriam experienced the shift that decades of diligence with exercise and following what we all used to believe was a "healthy diet" couldn't accomplish. And the best part? She did it without starving, without doing penance on a treadmill for perceived food sins, and without having every waking moment ruled by obsessive thoughts of food and diet-related numbers.

The approach outlined in *Breaking Free From Diet Prison: Common Sense Keto and Low Carb* will help you understand why and how to change your diet, whether you want to dive head-first into strict keto or make a more gradual entrance by cutting back on carbs little by little. There's no right or wrong way; there's only what suits you best. Miriam has left no stone unturned. She outlines the basics of how low carb diets work and equips you with the tools you need to be successful in the real world: shopping lists, tips for meal planning and food prep, and a step-by-step plan to take you from your current diet to one that shifts you from burning mostly carbs to burning mostly fat—and isn't that exactly what we want? To burn fat.

Miriam's writing is down-to-earth and conversational. You won't need a dictionary next to you while you read; she explains key concepts in plain English that's easy to understand and will be especially helpful for beginners to lower carb eating. This isn't an academic tome, but rather, a simple introduction to the whys and wherefores of low carb and keto, written in a tone that makes you feel like you're having coffee or tea with Miriam in her living room.

Something that makes *Breaking Free From Diet Prison: Common Sense Keto and Low Carb* especially unique is that it goes beyond the nuts and bolts of the food and addresses the psychology of habit change. This is a critical aspect, and one that's missing from most other keto books. After all, it doesn't matter how effective a diet is if mental and emotional roadblocks prevent you from following it. The sections on mindset are applicable no matter what diet you follow, keto or not, and are applicable for aspects of life far beyond diet altogether.

If you're looking to sift through the keto noise and find a way to move in the direction of lower carb eating—and to do it in a way that requires nothing you can't find at your neighborhood supermarket, no fancy gadgets and gizmos, no specialized and expensive keto products—let *Breaking Free From Diet Prison: Common Sense Keto and Low Carb* be your guide.

—Amy Berger, MS, CNS, Author of *End Your Carb Confusion, Alzheimer's Antidote,* and *The Stall Slayer*

PART ONE
INTRODUCTION AND WELCOME

The process of dieting is usually to do it and get it done. However, life and the way we live it, are never done. We try to diet – maybe even dozens of times – and then finally give up. I think it is because we never truly learn to trust what our body and mind are telling us.

For over 50 years I have searched for a way to diet and be done. "Be done" are the operative words here. On a diet, off a diet. Restrict, binge, give up, repeat. I was constantly on a hamster wheel, going nowhere, as best I could and as fast as I could. I could never stop, and I could never let my guard down. I could never find peace with food.

Finally, well into my sixties, I discovered keto and learned about insulin and about the influence that the food itself has on my mind and body, causing me to want more, crave more and stay hungry. While I successfully followed, taught and coached keto for over three years, establishing myself as Granny Keto, my life took a turn. I felt I needed to broaden my way of eating. My food lifestyle evolved as I learned to eat in a low carb way that still keeps insulin in check and the cravings and hunger at bay.

My own experience with keto came before my practice of low carb eating. This book, however, introduces low carb before going into depth with keto. In my practice I find that clients want to approach keto gradually rather than to jump right in. Starting them with low carbohydrate eating helps them on their journey and avoids the problems that immediate keto sometimes causes, such as the dreaded keto flu. Learning about low carb also helps clients avoid missteps because certain keto concepts are better understood when practiced slowly. However, if you are interested in jumping right to keto, you can skip to PART 3, GET THE KRAZINESS OUT OF KETO! so that you know what it's all about. But then please backtrack through PART 2, *GRANNY KETO TRANSITIONS PROGRAM™* so that you can learn more about the necessary elements for keto (low carbohydrate, adequate protein and high fat) and how to incorporate them into your lifestyle. In addition to guiding you with a slower approach to keto, this 5-step program can have its steps work independently of each other. Do you only want to get the sugar monkey off your back? Do you only need to go gluten free? *Granny Keto Transitions Program™* would be perfect for you!

PART 4 – MAKE LOW CARB AND KETO YOUR LIFESTYLE will help you with the most important parts of making this a true lifestyle so that you no longer have to weigh, measure or track your food. CHAPTER 13, DANCING WITH LOW CARB AND KETO, draws on my thirty years as a belly dance teacher and performer to turn those stage lessons into plate lessons! Part 4 also helps you better understand and work with your hunger scale and shows you how to keep this whole process simple.

Parts 5 and 6 – Meal Planning and Shopping and New Habits and Thoughts are your toolbox, packed with worksheets and lessons. These chapters will give you the guidance you need to turn your life around and break free from diet prison! No more confusion, shame or guilt. No more negative self-talk, aimless dreaming or running to satisfy a craving or urge. In these chapters you will find everything you will need, from meal planning and grocery shopping to goal setting and finding your reason for doing this.

My motto as a coach is "Nutritional coaching that meets you where you are and guides you to where you want to go." This book teaches you to live your life in a way that you can build your own road to where you want to go, just as I built mine. *Breaking Free From Diet Prison: Common Sense Keto and Low Carb* gives you three pillars to build this road. These pillars will give you healthy boundaries and keep you out of the breakdown lane. I teach you to dance all the way to finding and building a lifestyle that you and your family can enjoy. You will now have the tools to shift gears as you find necessary, but never get lost. The three pillars are:

- Education: the WHAT and WHY.

- Practical applications: the HOW.

- Mindfulness practices: the WHO (examining yourself and your habits and thoughts in a way you may never have before) and the WHEN (teaching you to move forward as you become ready).

Working with *Breaking Free From Diet Prison: Common Sense Keto and Low Carb* will help you to finally find peace with food. Yes, I said "working." Reading is good too, but I ask that you work with the practical applications and mindfulness practices to get the full benefit of what these three pillars offer you. If you do, I promise you will be off the diet roller coaster and free from diet prison. You may also want to look into my course: *Breaking Free From Diet Prison: The Roadmap to Low Carb and Keto Success™* (available at miriamhatoum.com) for "hands-on" work with these pillars.

These three pillars are here for you. They are the keys to your freedom. I am you. I used them and I found freedom. Now it's your turn.

CHAPTER ONE

MY STORY

I'm a wife, mother, and grandmother of two – and also a lifelong dieter. For years I was scolded by doctors who never believed I was following diet advice, a horrible cycle that started when I was just 13 years old! Listening to Gary Taubes's *Why We Get Fat and What to Do About It* was my lightbulb moment. For the first time, I realized that the food itself was keeping me fat all these years and it was not my fault. I began a ketogenic ("keto") diet immediately and never looked back. This book, however, is not just about keto. I am hoping to help you find some middle ground, using keto principles to eat a wise low carbohydrate diet or to eat keto in a way that melds with your lifestyle – no pills, shakes, gimmicks, weighing or measuring – just eating in a healthy way that supports weight loss in a way that feels good to you.

For myself, I enjoyed the freedom of keto (that's right – freedom even with all those food restrictions!) but I realized early on that keto is not for everyone, either because they don't want to do it or do not need to do it. My husband is one such person who is blessed with a great metabolism. I decided to widen my scope and create *Granny Keto Transitions Program: Five Steps to Keto*™. Because I was my own client, I found unique ways to make decisions about my eating protocol and to make true lifestyle changes. I used my experience of being a belly dance teacher to find methods to make permanent changes that stick. I am Miriam Hatoum, Granny Keto and Amira Jamal (my stage name) all rolled into one. I know with all my heart there is a way to dance through this instead of living in the prison of weighing, measuring and tracking every morsel of food.

What is your dieting history? Can you relate to mine?

Below is the long non-exhaustive list of diets I've tried. I am putting my list here so that you can see you are not alone. In doing keto, I realized, once and for all, that I never failed these diets. The diets failed me. Yes, I still needed personal work such as setting goals or sitting with urges, but, overall, after learning about insulin's effect on hunger and fat storage, I realized that the food itself was the major contributor driving me to eat. Have you done any – or ALL of these or MORE???

- At the age of 13, Mom took me to a doctor who put me on a calorie/exchange program AND put me on amphetamines – in 1965 I guess they were no big deal.

- At the age of 16, I was dropped off by my mom at Weight Watchers meetings.

- When I was in college, I put a fridge in my room and made a pudding out of Carnation Instant Breakfast, water and gelatin, and ate that instead of meals.

- Between the amphetamines and the Carnation Instant Breakfast pudding there must have been at least a dozen stupid (and dangerous) attempts to diet – it was, after all, the age of Twiggy.

- Stillman Diet – (precursor of Atkins®) – NOTHING but protein and vegetables. All I remember are cottage cheese and carrots.

- EVERY incarnation of Weight Watchers® – from the original (fish five times a week, liver and no-ketchup-only-mustard version) up through all the different POINTS systems. There have to have been no fewer than 20 different programs through the years, and I was on at least 18 of them.

- The Zone Diet

- CAD: Carbohydrate Addict Diet

- South Beach Diet

- Gluten Free Diet

- Glycemic Index and Glycemic Load diets

- (Medically supervised) Elimination Diet

- Tosca Reno's Clean Eating

- Joyce Meyers Eat and Stay Thin

- No S Diet

- Beck Diet

- Overeaters Anonymous

- 100 Days of Weight Loss

- Mark Hyman – Both Blood Sugar Diet and the Eat Fat Diet

- Volumetrics

- Never did juicing, but I did buy a Nutribullet thinking that a few of those recipes might "boost metabolism."

- Way-of-life sort-of diets: Mediterranean, Paleo, Primal (I actually draw on these now.)

- Calorie counting: My Fitness Pal, SparkPeople and Lose It (as well as paper and pencil during the dark ages).

- Suzanne Sommers (food combining)

- Any of the dozens of books with titles such as Think Yourself Thin, Thin From Within, etc.

- All sorts of exchange diets (American Heart, Diabetic, etc.)

- TOPS

- Eat This, Not That

- Hungry Girl Diet

- Tony Robbins: The Body You Deserve

- DASH Diet was supported by my workplace, so I looked, but did not follow.

- Positive Changes (Hypnosis, and by far the most-costly one even if I add up all my years and products at Weight Watchers.)

- The Slow Down Diet

- Intuitive Eating

- Mindful Eating

- Karly Pitman's Growing Human Kindness and Untangled programs

Not all these diets are off the mark, but they did not ring all the bells and blow all the whistles for me. In the past, I looked at all these attempts to diet as my failures. I have turned my thinking around and now see that it was just a matter of not succeeding, and that some of these diets had built-in problems because of the foods and methods, no matter how well-intentioned they were. I now no longer see myself as a failure, just attempts that did not work out, but which supplied the building blocks to bring me to where I am now. I am sure you have heard some of Thomas Edison's quotes, among them:

"I have not failed. I've just found 10,000 ways that won't work."

"Our greatest weakness lies in giving up. The most certain way to succeed is always to try just one more time."

"Results! Why, man, I have gotten a lot of results. I know several thousand things that won't work."

Bless you, Mr. Edison. I see I am not a failure nor were my hundreds of attempts at dieting in the 55+ years (!) I have been making them. They were merely steppingstones to finding what works, and to help me grow and mature. What I learned from trying all these diets is that the answer is within me and it is within you too. It is not just a matter of the foods themselves that we choose to eat, but also the emotions and feelings we have behind eating those foods. Let this book you hold in your hands, *Breaking Free From Diet Prison: Common Sense Keto and Low Carb*, meet you where you are in this journey and guide you to where you want to go. You can learn a joyous and sustainable way of eating without weighing, measuring or tracking your food. Aren't you ready for that?

I want to offer hope to people who share some of my dieting history. I do this by taking my coaching skills to the mat to help you eliminate negative thinking – whether the thinking is about you, the way you eat or any of the circumstances in your life. There is much more to my story in CHAPTER 8, MY ROAD TO KETO.

I work with clients who have been dieting for decades but who haven't given up. If you work with the three pillars, I promise you that this may – and probably will – be the last time you have to spend one more day on the diet roller coaster or in the diet prison of weighing, measuring and tracking every morsel of food that you eat. Whatever your story is, it can be a complicated one, especially when there are emotional issues and mindsets that keep us from following food protocols. It can be complicated if you are facing certain life situations – like being the filling for a sandwich: kids on one side and taking care of elderly parents on the other; retirement; loss of a spouse; or even a houseful of young children. And sometimes, really, it is just that you were never presented with the correct nutritional information, the tools showing you how to put things into practice or the guidance of how to wrap your mind around the changes you need to make. Now that you are holding this book in your hands, I will help you navigate these waters and find peace with food for perhaps the first time in your life.

My most challenging client was, and still is, myself, something that kept this book in a holding pattern for a long time. As I worked through many things, I realized that what I was learning and doing would help others to learn to lose weight in a way that would finally work. Just this morning at breakfast, I asked myself, "How would Granny Keto coach me in picking out just the right breakfast?"

If you are like me and tired of it all, you are ready to go on to read about what ketogenic and low carb eating is and the many ways of doing them. Maybe full keto doesn't float your boat at all, and you want a gradual shift in your eating habits. Maybe you are ready to commit to keto. Either way, *Breaking Free From Diet Prison: Common Sense Keto and Low Carb* is perfect for you!

GOOD TO KNOW...

Eating is a complex process. The food itself can drive eating as well as habits. There is neurobiological evidence that there are three neural pathways. Also, there are two regions of the brain (insula and the frontal operculum) that drive an elevated experience of reward (for some foods in some people) and a reduced ability to inhibit the drive to eat, and some combination of the two. The three neural pathways code for (1) the perceived importance of the food, (2) the rewarding sensation of actual eating and (3) the behavioral control based on consideration of short- and long-term consequences. These are related to the conditions of impulse control and delayed gratification, which are as much neurological and biological as they are a matter of habit. There is truth to saying that your brain lights up when it sees cookies and cake! It also explains why we turn to the same food and behaviors over and over again even though we hate doing it and know better. Stop beating yourself up! You are not "broken" you just have really good and strong pathways!

PART TWO
GRANNY KETO TRANSITIONS PROGRAM™

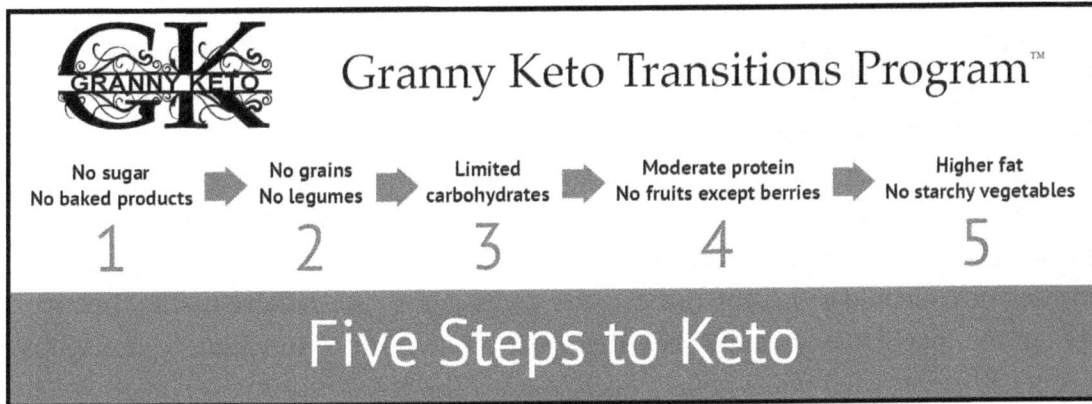

Granny Keto Transitions Program™

No sugar No baked products	No grains No legumes	Limited carbohydrates	Moderate protein No fruits except berries	Higher fat No starchy vegetables
1	2	3	4	5

Five Steps to Keto

I created this program when I was best known as Granny Keto. I have decided to keep it named as such even though I have moved on to being "just" Miriam Hatoum, coaching both keto and low carb. You will see other references to Granny Keto in this book, such as the Granny Keto Hybrid way to count your carbohydrates. My work as Granny Keto has inspired much of this book, my course and website (now miriamhatoum.com), but don't be confused. It's all me!

When working with clients on keto, I found I needed a way to honor my commitment "to provide nutritional coaching that meets you where you are and guides you to where you want to go." Some clients wanted to do keto after reading about its benefits in reversing type 2 diabetes, eliminating pre-diabetes, reducing fasting insulin, reversing NAFLD (non-alcoholic fatty liver disease) and helping to slow down, or stop, insulin resistance.

Many clients who had none of the above health issues still wanted to do keto to increase their overall health including improving HDL, lowering triglycerides, losing fat and building lean muscle mass. Among all my clients, whatever their motivation for wanting to do keto, I found two personalities: Those who love to jump into the deep end of a pool and those who would rather go in slowly, dipping one toe at a time. Because I am a "jump in the deep end" sort of gal, I really had to think through how to best help the toe-dippers.

I discovered a second thing that committed me to finding a way to develop this special program. Many people, especially those without pressing medical problems but who were interested in keto anyway, experienced almost immediate weight loss, better digestion, better sleep and improvement in general well-being before fully progressing through keto. I found that many clients were happy and feeling better just eliminating sugar and/or grains from their diets with no need or desire to go further.

Granny Keto Transitions Program™ was born! It is a program for those who want to slowly work up to being fully keto and also for those who are very happy eating low carb but need some guidance to pull it all together. You will see many references to keto in this program because that was the original intent of the program such as "eliminate starchy vegetables." As the program grew to accommodate my low carb clients, I added advice to perhaps limit something but not eliminate it. That is why you see references to both keto and low carb within one step.

As you read through the steps of this program, please do not feel rushed to jump through the steps like a game of hopscotch. Take your time. Make changes in your life and move forward slowly. Bring partners and family on board.

If you have decided in advance that you want to do keto immediately, it is okay to skip ahead to PART 3 to get to the Yes/No lists. However, please come back to this part of the book and program because it explains the reasons for each keto recommendation. I have found that understanding the reason you are being told to do something makes the change so much more lasting. The Appendix further outlines popular keto approaches. Regardless of your initial intention, you may find that keto is not something you want to jump into right away. The TRANSITIONS program gives you a way to slowly work your way up.

Granny Keto Transitions Program™ contains very detailed lists of sugars, grains, legumes and rice that you will need to know about in order to be successful on keto and low carb. It is an eye-opener to read this list of carbohydrates that are in our everyday diets. You may not have thought twice about the carbohydrates in foods such as fruits, seeds, nuts and dairy. Each step also includes a mindfulness practice that you won't want to miss.

You will find that some key points circle back on themselves and that there is some repetition among the chapters. The reasons for this are twofold: First, you may be skipping between parts or chapters as you decide whether or not to work the *Granny Keto Transitions Program*™ as a low carb approach or to jump into the deep end and immediately go full keto. There is information that you need with either approach. I want to make sure you don't miss it. Second, it is important to hear a few things more than once, so the repetition is by design!

I find that *Granny Keto Transitions Program*™ enables me to honor that commitment of "nutritional coaching that meets you where you are and guides you to where you want to go." I am very proud of it and honored to share it with you.

Chapter Two

Introduction to Granny Keto Transitions Program™

Being fully keto does fabulous healthy things for your body. You not only will lose weight, but it will usually put type 2 diabetes into remission, reduce your insulin needs for type 1 diabetes, reverse insulin resistance, reverse non-alcoholic fatty liver disease, lower blood pressure and so much more. This program will give you a starting point to go step-by-step to keto or guide you into a comfortable low carb eating plan. This program allows you to land and stay on any step you like! You do not even have to go as far as keto – you can take one step at a time in combination with, or separate from, any of the other steps.

If you know you want to follow keto but are totally new or unfamiliar it, I invite you to skip to Chapter 9, Understanding Keto, so that you will gain a better understanding why the progression of the steps in *Granny Keto Transitions Program*™ are laid out the way they are. You may decide to move toward becoming fully keto, but there are many reasons why this might not be your ultimate goal:

- Maybe your metabolism is fine, and you are not the slightest bit overweight, but you have a sugar demon that you cannot get off your back.

- Maybe you have a child or family member with diabetes, and you want to be a good role model and show that there is indeed life without sugar.

- Maybe you have tried over and over again to lose weight but always return to old eating habits and weight gain. This program will teach you that it is possible that the food itself can cause cravings and overeating.

- Maybe you or someone in your family needs to eat gluten-free (or totally grain-free) and you would like guidance with meal planning and with shopping lists to accommodate this change.

- Maybe you have fine control with sugar, grains and baked goods, but you want to learn how to incorporate more lower carb eating into your lifestyle.

- Maybe you have done your research and you are ready to begin keto, but you don't know where or how to begin. Working with the steps of *Granny Keto Transitions Program*™ will be just what you need!

Here is a bird's eye view of *Granny Keto Transitions Program*™. You can work all steps starting anywhere on the staircase or just go as far as you want to go! CHAPTERS 3 through 7 go into detail for each step.

STEP 1: ELIMINATE SUGAR AND BAKED PRODUCTS

These two are together because although you might be able to give up your sugar fixes, it does you no good if you then eat bread or even a sugar-free pastry. Start here with having no "outright" sugar (i.e., sugar in your coffee, candy, honey in your tea, etc.). At this step you will learn that fruit is fructose and the fiber in it does not mitigate that fact. Yes, a whole fruit hits your bloodstream more slowly than juice because of the fiber, but a whole fruit is still fructose, glucose and sucrose, and those are all sugar. At the very least, please limit your fruits to no more than one or two servings a day. An entire fruit bowl is not necessarily a good alternative to a candy bar!

This first step requires awareness. Did you know that there are many names for hidden sugar and the list increases annually? You may know that high fructose corn syrup (HFCS) is on the list, but as you start to read labels (which is essential at this step!) you will learn to identify all of them. The list is in CHAPTER 3. You will also learn about the fact that all carbohydrates are essentially sugar and even at this step you are encouraged to limit, or at least be aware of, your intake of other foods such as grains, legumes and starchy vegetables.

STEP 2: ELIMINATE GRAINS AND LEGUMES

This is the biggest step after getting the sugar out of your diet. Keep TRANSITIONS STEP 1 intact if you are moving towards a keto lifestyle. However, if you are looking to stay here for a while and eat more of a Paleo or Primal lifestyle you are allowed honey and pure maple syrup back into your diet. Be forewarned: Something like a Paleo banana bread made with honey and bananas is not only dangerous for insulin levels and sugar cravings but does not help you at all if your ultimate goal is keto.

Just like with the list of hidden sugars (CHAPTER 3) it is important to know what grains are. Most of you would recognize wheat, corn and barley as grains but there are so many more. In CHAPTER 4 there is a rather complete list of grains, rice and legumes. Included in the grains list are "pseudograins" which come from the seeds of broadleaf plants and not thin-leaf cereal plants. These grains do not contain gluten, so if your main goal is to be gluten-free, these grains (and rice) are okay at TRANSITIONS STEP 2, but they are not allowed on keto, where your total carbs for the day come to less than what is in one cup of rice! Also, all grains have inflammatory properties so if you are on a mission to heal your gut, you may not want to eat anything from that list, whether or not you ever go to fully keto.

STEP 3: EATING LOW CARB

This might be a great step for you to land on and stay a while. This is the step where you will become aware of the carbohydrate counts of fruits, vegetables, dairy, nuts, grains and legumes. If you have chosen to go gluten-free only and have kept some of the foods in Step 2 in your diet, this step will be an eye-opener for you. The Standard American Diet (often referred to as SAD) can be 400 to 500 or more carbohydrates a day even if you are not overeating or bingeing. These carbohydrates add up – one meal will usually have 100 or more carbohydrates! By the time your day is done with three meals and perhaps two to three snacks, you are easily looking at that SAD amount of 500 carbs or more.

STEP 4: MODERATE PROTEIN AND NO FRUIT EXCEPT BERRIES

(FOR LOW CARB YOU WILL BE LIMITING FRUITS, NOT ELIMINATING THEM.)

I would have started keto six months sooner than I did if I did not hear "No fruit except for berries." I said, "No way am I ever giving up fruit. Are they crazy?" But then I started learning, opening my mind and accepting the truth.

There are a few issues with fruit. Let's just start with the pure sugar and carb content of fruits. If you are going to be fully keto you will be restricting your carbohydrates. However, there is a more serious concern with fruit that goes beyond counting carbohydrates. Fructose, the sugar in fruit, cannot be used by your cells for energy. Fructose goes directly to the liver to be metabolized and can cause a fatty liver which is linked to early death, diabetes and heart disease. Fructose also makes you more insulin resistant. It causes your triglycerides to go up, it increases inflammation and has a terrible effect on your cholesterol. Berries, by contrast, in moderation (about ½ cup) not only have much less sugar but their glycemic load is also low, meaning they will very slowly, if at all, raise a person's blood glucose level.

Protein is the building block of cells and muscles, and it is essential for brain function and to heal cuts and wounds. However, the body "recycles" much of its proteins and we do not need to consume large quantities to have a healthy body. However, we do not have to be afraid to consume protein. The new face of keto is that if you are hungry add a little more protein instead of fat. This is especially true for older women. It has been found that the older you are, the less efficiently you process protein. This means that a little more protein than previously thought is healthy.

In TRANSITIONS STEP 4 you will be encouraged to eliminate fruits except for berries, and to learn how to moderate your protein intake in healthy and creative ways. Again, you do not have to worry about too much protein, but you will learn what it means to moderate it. If you have chosen a low carb eating style then you will not be eliminating fruit, but you will get the information to make informed decisions about limiting it. This step is the springboard to the final TRANSITIONS step that will get you to your goal of being fully keto.

STEP 5: EAT HIGHER FAT AND ELIMINATE STARCHY VEGETABLES
(FOR LOW CARB YOU WILL BE LIMITING, NOT ELIMINATING, STARCHY VEGETABLES.)

You have arrived at the final step of being FULL KETO. Congratulations!! In this step you will have the final piece of the puzzle – eating higher fat, and your final elimination: starchy vegetables. If you have chosen to eat in a low carb way rather than keto, you do not have to eliminate starchy vegetables, but you will learn to moderate them.

The MYTH (known as the Diet-Heart hypothesis) is that fats (especially saturated fats) are bad for you. As a matter of fact, they serve very important functions such as building cell walls, and helping with mineral absorption and mineral conversion. For instance, the fat-soluble vitamins A, D, E, and K are called fat-soluble for a reason! If you eat low-fat or no-fat, you will not get the full benefit of these vitamins. Furthermore, fat is the one macronutrient that has little to no effect on your insulin, so it is the perfect food to add to your meals for satiety, flavor and enjoyment. The takeaway is to not skimp on real fats! TRANSITIONS STEP 5 will walk you through adding fats to your meal and will also give you the complete picture of what your plate should look like. You will have a better understanding of the proportions of each macronutrient (carbohydrate, protein and fat) so that you can begin to eat a well-formulated ketogenic (keto) diet or a healthy low carb diet.

You cannot eat high fat *and* high carbohydrate. This is dangerous to your heart health. Therefore, even though I stated that you can stay at any step, I would not pick this one out of the hat and stay here separate from the other steps. Because TRANSITIONS STEP 5 is the final step to being fully keto, it pulls the whole picture together and you cannot live it as a fragment keeping both carbohydrates and fat intake high.

Because now you understand that you can find satiety and satisfaction with fat, it is the perfect time to take those potatoes and carrots off your plate. You are ready now ready to become fully keto. If you have decided to stay on a low carb path, then you will be more generous with your daily carbohydrate intake, allowing you to consume starchy vegetables.

THIS IS THE TOP STEP: FULL KETO

CHAPTER 9, UNDERSTANDING KETO, will give you a thorough explanation of what keto will look like as you come to the top step of *Granny Keto Transitions Program*™.

The biggest shift you will have to make, beyond what foods you are eating, is your mindset. Going keto is an entire paradigm shift, not a diet. You have to have a strong enough WHY (see CHAPTER 19, YOUR WHY) to see you through this. You need to do this for health! You will lose weight, of course, but this is a whole new way of eating for you, and you must be able to sustain it. That is where your WHY comes in. You have to be strong not because keto is difficult (actually it will become easier and easier, I promise) but because health is a lifetime commitment.

Once you decide whether you are planning to become fully keto you may still need to work on the "bones" (eat this and not that type of thing, planning family meals, outings, work lunches, etc.). But the most helpful thing is to wrap your mind around this paradigm shift and to realize you are worth it. You are worth the hard work and the health that it brings. Both keto and low carb are wonderful ways to bring your body and your mind into alignment with health. In truth, staying on TRANSITIONS STEP 1, STEP 2 or STEP 3 alone will bring your body and your mind into alignment with health. The work of going through TRANSITIONS STEP 4 and STEP 5 to get to full keto will be worth it as well if your body needs "super help" to get your weight down and your metabolism humming!

The rest of PART 2 goes into each of the steps of *Granny Keto Transitions Program*™ in more detail.

GOOD TO KNOW…

Insulin acts like a key to let glucose into cells for use as energy. When everything runs well, the food you eat is broken down into glucose, the glucose enters your blood stream and the pancreas is signaled to release insulin. Insulin helps this glucose enter the body's cells so that it can be used as energy, and it signals the liver to store any extra glucose for later use. When the glucose enters cells and the levels in the bloodstream decrease, insulin is signaled to decrease as well. When you are insulin resistant and a lot of glucose enters the blood stream, the pancreas pumps out more and more insulin in an effort to get glucose into cells. After a time, cells stop responding to all that insulin and that is known as "insulin resistance." Eventually the glucose in the blood keeps rising (which is type 2 diabetes). Keto is a wonderful way to eat to reverse insulin resistance and, as a matter of fact, many doctors report that patients with type 2 diabetes are able to come off their medication. Even taking smaller steps such as those in STEPS 1 and 2 of *Granny Keto Transitions Program*™, might be all you need to achieve a reversal of insulin resistance.

CHAPTER THREE

STEP 1: ELIMINATE SUGAR AND BAKED GOODS

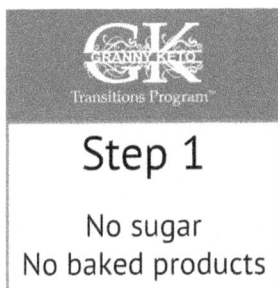

Step 1

No sugar
No baked products

Take this step as either a stand-alone step or the first step in a series of steps (whether or not you ever go fully keto). TRANSITIONS STEP 1 might be your only step and that is perfectly fine. I did a sugar "detox" program years ago – before I even heard of the word keto – just to get the sugar monkey off my back. It was even before I was concerned about pre-diabetes. I did not know about what I now call the Triad Connection: Insulin – Blood Sugar – Carbohydrate Consumption. As a stand-alone step, STEP 1 of *Granny Keto Transitions Program*™ will put you in good stead for your physical health. Just by cutting out sugar and baked goods you will get enough carbohydrates out of your system to help you feel better because doing so will reduce inflammation and lower your insulin levels. It will also help your mental health. I know there were many prongs to my sugar monkey. I felt as though there was no hope because I was always hungry and always craving sweet foods no matter how hard I dieted. I felt as though there was a defect in me. I didn't know to blame the sugar itself! As the veil of sugar cravings was lifted, I felt better physically and mentally. I call it a veil because it wasn't always that the candy reached out its talons and grabbed me by the throat. It was often subtler – just that I was never satisfied and always looking for more. And more. And more.

These two – no sugar and no baked goods – are put together in one step because although you might be able to give up sugar, it does you no good if you then eat bread or something like a sugar-free pastry. Start here with no "outright" sugar (i.e., sugar in your coffee, candy, honey in your tea, etc.) and sugar (by any name) in processed food. As stated in CHAPTER 2, INTRODUCTION TO *GRANNY KETO TRANSITIONS PROGRAM*™, please be aware that fruit is also sugar. The fiber in it does not mitigate that fact. Yes, a whole fruit will hit your blood stream more slowly than juice because of the fiber in an intact fruit, but a whole fruit is still mainly fructose, glucose and sucrose – all sugars. At the very least, please limit your fruits to one or two servings a day. An entire fruit bowl is not necessarily a good alternative to a candy bar! This first step requires additional awareness. Did you know that there are many names for sugar, and that manufacturers add to the list yearly? You may know that High Fructose Corn Syrup (HFCS) is on the list but as you start to read labels you will learn to identify all of them. Every year new renditions of sugar are invented, so look at this list as an extensive one, but not necessarily an exhaustive one.

Acesulfame potassium (AS) (Ace-K)

Agave

Agave nectar

Aspartame (AS)

Barbados sugar

Barley malt

Beet sugar

Blackstrap molasses

Brown sugar

Buttered syrup

Cane juice

Cane juice crystals

Cane sugar

Caramel

Carob syrup

Castor sugar

Coconut nectar

Coconut sugar/crystals

Confectioner's sugar

Corn syrup

Corn syrup solids

Crystalline fructose

Cyclamate (AS)

Date sugar

Date syrup

Dates

Demerara sugar

Dextran

Dextrose

Diastatic malt

Erythritol

Glucose solids

Golden sugar

Golden syrup

Grape sugar

High-fructose corn syrup

Icing sugar

Invert sugar

Lactitol (SA)

Lactose

Levulose

Light brown sugar

Luo han guo (monk fruit) (SA)

Maltitol (SA)

Malt syrup

Maltodextrin

Maltose

Mannitol (SA)

Maple syrup

Molasses

Monk fruit (SA)

Muscovado

Organic raw sugar

Palm sugar

Panocha

Raw sugar

Refiner's sugar

Rice syrup

Saccharin (AS)

Sorbitol (SA)

Sorghum syrup

Stevia (SA)

Evaporated cane juice	Sucralose (AS)
Florida crystals	Sucrose
Fructose	Tagatose
Fruit Juice	Treacle
Fruit juice concentrate	Turbinado sugar
Galactose	Yellow sugar
Glucose	Xylitol (SA)

*SA: Sugar Alternative (from natural sources {although it might be highly processed}, no calories)

*AS: Artificial Sweetener

Whether you use artificial sweeteners (AS on the list) at this (or any) point is a personal decision. Sugar alternatives (SA on the list) fare somewhat better in the research, although some of them tend to come with their own set of problems such as digestive issues. I encourage you to research and find resources that will help you decide. Be aware that if you find ten articles or studies on the subject, five will say it is harmful to consume them, and the other five will say it is not harmful to consume them. That is why you will have to make your own decision. Many people, however, find that their weight loss will stall with some sugar substitutes, even the natural sugar alternatives (not full laboratory chemicals) with no calories. Some of the science behind this is that although artificial sweeteners may not raise your blood sugar and they are zero calories, they might, for some people, raise insulin levels. Insulin is a fat-storage hormone so anything that raises it, independent of blood sugar, will cause a stall in weight loss.

Furthermore, some people will find that they cannot get rid of their sugar cravings while consuming anything sweet, whether it is a natural sweet (like fruit) or artificially sweet (like sugar-free Jell-O®). However, it is better to follow a sugar-elimination program than not, and sometimes it will be the difference between feeling you have to give up your coffee thus not even starting the program, or having one or two cups of coffee with a packet of Splenda® while you continue to move forward. That being said, it is not a license to eat unlimited quantities of sugar-free this and sugar-free that (sugar-free popsicles, sugar-free puddings and sugar-free Jell-O®, for instance). You must get rid of the sugar cravings. Sugar in any form (even artificial sugar) begets sugar cravings. However, a little bit of non-caloric sweetener might help you get "over the hump" and help you find success in giving up sugar, and that is what is important. It is more important to have a bridge than not try to cross the river at all! As you become secure in your new way of eating and your tastes change, it will become easier to give up even artificial sugar. Be honest. A packet of Splenda® or Sweet and Low® in a coffee is not the same as packing your kitchen with all things sugar-free!

One artificial sweetener, Acesulfame Potassium (sometimes referred to as Ace-K), found in a lot of artificially sweetened items, is worth noting. Many people have an insulin response to this sweetener. As stated above, insulin is the fat-storage hormone, and thus, high insulin leads to the inability to lose weight because insulin locks the fat into your fat cells. If you MUST drink diet sodas, look for Acesulfame Potassium on the label and if your brand has it as its sweetener, you may want to consider switching to some brand that does not have it. You can also start to cut back such as having one can of an Ace-K offender instead of a whole liter bottle. Anecdotally this also happens to some people with stevia even though it is considered a "natural" sweetener. When people say they lost a lot of weight by stopping the diet soda, sometimes they lose weight because they got rid of the type of sweetener that causes an insulin spike for them. This is not the same as a blood sugar spike, which is why these artificial sweeteners pass muster as a diet drink: they are still zero calories. Just as a coffee with Splenda® may help you get through your day, so may diet soda. Just be aware that if you are doing "everything right" but are consuming a lot of artificial sweeteners or sugar alternatives, be open to the fact it might be your choice of sweetener even if the calorie count is zero.

Fruit is addressed more fully in TRANSITIONS STEP 4. In STEP 1, I suggest that you limit your fruit intake to no more than one or two per day. You would be further helping yourself if you keep your choices to fresh fruits and stay away from dried fruits. For example, ½ cup of dried dates is 65 carbohydrates while ½ cup of fresh grapefruit or melon is about 8 carbohydrates. I know that you may not be interested in counting carbohydrates at this point, but it is important to know that once you take out the fiber (which amounts to very little in some fruits) the rest is fructose, sucrose and glucose – all sugar! Fructose is the main culprit for a lot of metabolic problems. This is because it is metabolized only by the liver and cannot be used by other cells in your body. Therefore, the liver has to work overtime to get rid of it. Eating bowls of fresh fruit does you no favor even if you cut out other sugars.

You will have a much harder time curbing your sugar cravings if you are consuming any amount of sugar, even if it is in the form of fruit. I am not saying no fruit, but again, please limit it. And, if you cannot do without, at least do not eat dried fruits and limit tropical fruits such as banana, mango, pineapple and papaya. These are loaded with sugar compared to fruits such as apples, berries and melons in the same quantities.

Let's now talk baked goods. Let's face it, a box of cookies is not the only place where we are going. I think you know that. I am talking bread.

That's right. B-R-E-A-D.

"I can't give up bread." Yes, you can. And I am talking ALL bread here – even keto bread made with almond and coconut flours…for now. I want you to get bread out of your system, not look for substitutes. By the time you reach TRANSITIONS STEP 5, you may have keto bread if you want to. However, as with the sweeteners, some people will never rid themselves of cravings if all they do is substitute one type of bread for another.

A very meaningful quote for me is Frank Ocean's, *"Whatever you do, never run back to what broke you."* When you cut out sugar and wheat flour, a lot of the physical cravings will subside, but if sweets and baked goods are triggers for you, you will have no relief from "head cravings" if you continue to eat all the foods that you were out of control with in the first place. For example, what happens if you allow yourself keto versions of bread while you are still at TRANSITIONS STEP 1 (because you don't consider keto baked goods "real" baked goods) or TRANSITIONS STEP 2 (because keto breads contain no grain)? What happens is that when you are looking for bread you won't have learned to tell yourself NO, and you will reach for what is available. Trust me on this: NO BREAD OF ANY KIND.

"OMG," you ask, "how do I take lunch to work if I can't take a sandwich?" Again, think a little bit outside the box. Take a filling with you (deli meat, tuna salad, etc.) and bring lettuce (not iceberg: it is too stiff) and make yourself rollups. (A side note: I have found from experience that any lettuce rollup made with a mayo filling gets soggy in transit. Bring the lettuce and filling separately and make your rollups when you are going to eat them.) "Can I have low carb wraps?" NO, you cannot. They are baked goods and the same as bread. Be creative. Use lettuce or cheese rollups or be even more creative and get out of the sandwich habit. "HUH? No sandwich for lunch?" Well, first of all, anything travels without bread – use baggies and small containers and bring a fork. There are tons of grab-and-go foods too: Beef jerky, hard boiled eggs, salami and cheese (slices or rollups), cut veggies and ranch dip. Come on – you didn't get overweight by not understanding the concept of how to get food into your mouth. YOU DO NOT NEED BREAD.

"But what about sopping up gravy?" You are ONLY on TRANSITIONS STEP 1. At this point you can still have gravy (made without flour) and rice and even mashed potatoes. (Oh, this sounds so wrong to me, but I am willing to say let's start with just no sugar and no baked goods.) YOU DO NOT NEED BREAD.

Can you do me a favor though? Limit yourself with other "starchy" things: ONE potato per day – and please make it a sweet potato more often than a white potato if you must have one. Have ONE cup of rice or ONE cup of pasta or ONE cup of corn per day (not per meal). And remember, a cup is about the size your fist. Measure these things out the first dozen or so times you eat them but then you can begin to eyeball the quantity and probably be spot on with it. You want to make this as much of a comfortable lifestyle as possible. Fill up on non-starchy vegetables (cooked or raw), fresh salads and non-cream soups. Enjoy proteins, plain or with sauces made with no added sugar.

This is not a cookbook, and you can find plenty of these recipes anywhere. But to get you thinking, how do these sound to you?

- Chicken cacciatore or chicken Parmesan (made without breading on the chicken)
- Garlic-butter sautéed mushrooms (nothing but the butter, garlic and mushrooms)
- Fried rice (using riced cauliflower – it's actually good)

- Buffalo chicken wings (find any buffalo sauce without sugar and go to town)
- Bacon and pepperoni "crackers" (a strip of bacon cut into thirds or quarters, or small pepperoni slices baked until crisp)

Not a piece of bread or grain of sugar in sight.

Let me talk a bit about why I am also asking you to limit other starches as well (potatoes, pasta, rice, corn, etc.) even though they are allowed at this step. Without getting all science-y there are a few things that are important to know. Especially if you are looking at this for weight loss, it is good to understand that you are not unhealthy because you are fat. You are fat because you are unhealthy. Insulin is behind weight gain and stubborn fat. Too much insulin is what is unhealthy. Carbohydrates (regardless of their source: starch or sugar) feed insulin. Simply put, all carbohydrates are sugar, whether they are simple or complex, and most break down into the simple sugar glucose in your blood stream. No, a potato does not turn into a piece of chocolate cake, but the base components are practically identical. Once carbohydrates hit your digestive system, liver, pancreas and bloodstream, your body, and thus insulin, perceive and manage them usually as the simple sugar, glucose. Once you are eating keto (the top step) you will no longer be flooding your body with sugar, but for now, it is okay that you just START to stop flooding your body with sugar. Just as sugar begets sugar cravings, because all carbohydrates are essentially sugar in your body, carbohydrates beget sugar cravings. Even if you have no intention of going all the way to the keto step, why torture yourself with cravings when you are working so hard on Transitions Step 1? There is more on this subject in Chapter 9, Understanding Keto.

This can be an easy and doable lifestyle. Just don't eat sugar directly or processed food containing sugar (or any name for sugar). Don't eat bread or other baked goods even if they are "sugar-free." If you do this, then the ONLY limits (and limited measuring until you get used to eyeballing the quantity) you have are other carbohydrates such as fruit and starchy vegetables like peas and corn (which is actually a grain but is often grouped with vegetables). Root vegetables like potatoes, carrots and beets should also be limited. The root (which is the portion of the vegetable you eat) is the underground storehouse for the sugar that provides energy to grow the green tops. Also limit pasta, rice and foods that may be made with flour that are not baked goods, such as gravies and creamed soups. Be honest with yourself. I don't want to give you enough rope to hang yourself, but I do want to give you enough rope to start to feel some sense of accomplishment and also have a sense of self-efficacy, maybe for the first time in your life.

What is self-efficacy? It is a PERSONAL judgment (not someone else judging you) about how well you can do something in the face of effort and obstacles. It means that you will start to feel good about yourself and, because my favorite word in this step seems to be "begets," I will say that success begets success. Your belief (and results) about being able to follow this step begets further beliefs that you can follow this – and any further – step!

Mindfulness Practice

Mindfulness practices are included with each step. For this step, just put your fork down between bites (or put the food down, for instance if you are eating a rollup). You probably eat way too fast anyway and because you may be harboring some anxiety with this process you will find that the food will be gone even more quickly without even realizing that you ate it! Also, it is true that it takes about 20 minutes for the full signal to hit your brain. The science-y explanation: It normally takes 20 minutes for food to get from the stomach to the ileum in the small intestine. The ileum secretes the gut hormone, PYY, which is responsible for making you feel full. That is why it is better to eat slowly, and this will take care of "How do I know I am full?" This is a question and skill we examine in the mindfulness practice in Transitions Step 4 (Chapter 6) and again in Part 4, Making Low Carb and Keto a Lifestyle.

P.S. YOU DON'T NEED BREAD!

Good to Know...

A Connecticut College study found that "Even though we associate significant health hazards in taking drugs like cocaine and morphine, high-fat/high-sugar foods may present even more of a danger because of their accessibility and affordability." As with many other studies, it has been found that sugar activates the opiate receptors in our brain and affects the reward center, which leads to compulsive behavior, despite the negative consequences. This is why people feel addicted to sugar and baked goods. When one cookie leads to the entire box and you feel out of control, you can be assured it is not in your head. It is a very real thing. You are not damaged. You are human.

CHAPTER FOUR

STEP 2: ELIMINATE GRAINS AND LEGUMES

Step 2

No grains
No legumes

Okay ladies and gentlemen – hold on to your hats. This is the biggest step after getting the sugar out of your diet. You must keep STEP 1 intact if you are moving towards a keto lifestyle. If you are looking to stay here for a while but eat more of a "Paleo" or "Primal" diet you are allowed back honey and pure maple syrup. However, as I said earlier, be forewarned that something like a Paleo banana bread made with honey and bananas not only is dangerous for insulin levels and sugar cravings, but it also does not help you at all if your ultimate goal is keto. Wanting to go gluten-free and/or trying to heal gut issues associated with grains and legumes makes this a valuable stand-alone step.

Similar to the list of hidden sugars it is helpful to know what is considered a grain. Most of you would recognize wheat, corn and barley as grains but there are so many more. Also included in this list are "pseudograins" which come from the seeds of broadleaf plants and not the thin-leaf cereal plants. Pseudograins do not contain gluten, so if your main goal is to be gluten-free, these grains (and rice) are okay in TRANSITIONS STEP 2. They are not allowed on keto where your total carbs for the day come to less than what is in one cup of rice! They also have inflammatory properties. If you are on a mission to heal your gut, I urge you to refrain from eating anything from the grains list, whether or not your ultimate goal is to go fully keto.

Rice is also a grain (although we often put it in its own category). As with grains, rice is a known source (or aggravation) of inflammation, auto-immune diseases and leaky gut. Rice is allowed if you are gluten intolerant or gluten sensitive, but because of the high carbohydrate count of rice (whatever kind) most people will stay away from it on keto, although you can have it if you are eating low carb, as long as you pay attention to the quantity you are eating.

Legumes have the same inflammatory properties as grains and rice, and also contain phytic acid and lectins which can interfere with absorption of nutrients. There are some methods of cooking and preparing legumes and other grains (such as pre-soaking or sprouting) that can somewhat mitigate this, but again, as with rice, the carbohydrate count of this food makes this a category you may want to limit or avoid even if you are not eating keto.

My on-line course *Breaking Free From Diet Prison: The Roadmap to Low Carb and Keto Success*™ (at miriamhatoum.com) goes into much further detail on inflammation, leaky gut and gluten intolerance.

GRAINS AND SOME GRAIN PRODUCTS

"Finished" items such as pasta, cake, cookies, etc. are not on this list. The items on the list are things you might come across on labels, in recipe ingredients and on restaurant menus that you might not immediately recognize as being in the family of grains.

Amaranth (pseudograin)	Oat bran
Atta flour	Oat groats
Barley	Oats
Barley flakes	Orzo
Barley grits	Panko (made from wheat)
Buckwheat (pseudograin)	Pearl/Pearled barley
Buckwheat grits	Polenta
Buckwheat groats/unroasted buckwheat	Popcorn
Bulgur wheat	Pot/scotch barley
Corn	Quick cooking oats/quick oatmeal
Corn flour/meal	Quinoa (pseudograin)
Couscous	Rice (see separate rice list)
Cracked rye	Rolled oats/old fashioned oatmeal
Durham wheat	Rye
Einkorn	Rye berries
Emmer	Seitan (made from wheat)
Farro	Semolina
Freekeh	Sorghum
Graham	Spelt
Grain alcohol (whiskey, bourbon, scotch)	Spelt berries
Hominy	Spelt flakes
Hulled barley/Barley groats	Steel-cut oats/Irish oatmeal
Instant oats/instant oatmeal	Teff
Kasha/roasted buckwheat	Triticale
Khorasan (Kamut)	Triticale berries

Malt whiskey

Malts

Matzo meal

Muesli (made from oats or wheat)

Millet (pseudograin)

Montina™ Flour

Triticale flakes

Udon noodles

Wheat

Wheat berries

Wheat nuts

RICE

Arborio

Basmati

Bhutanese red

Black japonica

Brown

Calrose

Camargue red rice/riz rouge

Carnaroli

Forbidden/black forbidden rice

Instant

Jasmine

Kalijira/kala jeera

Long grain

Medium grain

Parboiled/converted

Paella (Calasparra, Valencia, Patna)

Popcorn (basmati & American long-grain rice)

Purple sticky

Short grain

Sticky/glutinous/sweet/mochi

Sushi

White

Wild

LEGUMES (BEANS)

Adzuki beans

Anasazi beans

Black beans/black turtle beans

Black-eyed peas

Borlotti/cranberry/roman

Butter beans

Cannellini beans

Christmas lima bean/chestnut lima

Corona beans

Fava beans/broad beans

Lima beans

Lupini beans

Marrow beans

Moth beans

Mung beans

Navy beans

Pigeon pea

Pink beans

Pinto beans

Red beans/small red beans

Flageolet beans	Rice beans
Garbanzo beans/chickpeas	Scarlet runner beans
Desi/Bengal Gram	Soybean/soya bean
Chana dal (split)	Spanish tolosana beans
Great northern beans	Split peas: green, yellow
Kidney beans	Tepary beans
Lentils: green, red, yellow, brown	Urad

The peanut, which is actually a legume and not a nut, is not on this list. It is allowed on a keto diet and so I allow it here. Just as with artificial sweeteners, it is your personal decision whether to eat them. Peanuts cause inflammation for some people. If you have peanuts one night and your hands or feet (or any other body part) feel stiff the next day, then it is probably due to the peanuts. However, inflammation does not just hit your joints. Inflammation can be in the gut, your arteries or in other parts of your system. Furthermore, some peanuts are susceptible to fungus. Eating dry-roasted Valencia peanuts will soften this blow because they are grown in drier climates that are naturally resistant to the fungus. With the inflammation and chance of fungus (which your body might also be very sensitive to) it becomes a personal decision whether to have them at all. Also be aware of the fat, protein and carbohydrate counts before you grab a handful for a snack. If you eat peanut butter eat it dry roasted – no oil or sugars added. Some grocery stores may let you grind your own.

Now that you are not eating sugar, grains, legumes, bread or any other baked goods, you will find yourself eating very few processed foods. GOOD! You will get used to it. You didn't think you would survive the no-bread rule, did you? And yet, here you are.

As I said earlier, if your goal is to just go gluten-free at this point you can have the pseudograins (amaranth, buckwheat, millet, quinoa), rice and legumes. But again, as with the advice in Step 1 to limit starchy vegetables and fruit, I would ask that you get used to limiting these as well, whether or not your goal is to go fully keto. I say this because these foods are very high in carbohydrates, and for general health it is important to keep your carbohydrates in check. ALL of them turn into glucose in your system and if you have read about keto, you will know that being a sugar-burner is less desirable than being a fat-burner. Not only that, but your overall health is susceptible to high insulin and inflammation, both of which occur if you do not keep your carbs – gluten-free or not – in check.

In terms of meal planning and recipes without grains and legumes, I assume you are here because you are looking for a way to help your body back to health. Did you survive meals with no bread? Did you manage to bring a work lunch that wasn't a sandwich? Did you find grab-and-go snacks like salami, hard-boiled eggs, and cheese? GREAT! Now let's move on from there! This is where we get into meal planning for the family. Make proteins and vegetables that you will enjoy. At this point you can still have starchy vegetables like potatoes and carrots, but please limit them!

If your family is looking for rice or pasta with a meal go ahead and make it and serve it to them. You can replace these starches with a small sweet potato or serving of roasted root vegetable, or avoid a starch altogether! Honestly, if you serve full and interesting meals to your family, they shouldn't be balking at the lack or reduction of bread, grains and legumes. Or maybe they will. You can still serve these things, but you have to have your own sense of what is important. Look out for your own best interests, whether or not you have support from friends and family. (See more about meal planning for the family in PART 5.)

If you work away from home and you need to pack lunches, you can keep taking what you made when you did Step 1. Need some variety? This is where you might look at some recipes that travel well and with or without needing to be reheated in a microwave. For lunches that do not have to be refrigerated or heated you can stick with things like:

- Salami and cheese with salad or crunchy vegetables like celery, radishes and bell peppers.

- Sliced deli meat – any type. Check that it does not have sugar – usually roast beef, turkey or chicken breast, pastrami, mortadella and corned beef work well. Roll the meat up in lettuce leaves or a cheese wrap.

- Egg or tuna salad. We are not watching fat. Use enough real mayonnaise to be satisfying. Unless you are making your own mayonnaise watch the bottled stuff. Most have sugar. If you use full-fat mayonnaise, there is less chance of sugar. There are some lovely avocado-oil mayonnaise products, and sugar is so far down on the ingredient list that the carb count for a serving is zero. Do not use mayonnaise products and other dressings that are mostly all chemicals!

Try your deli meat with ranch dressing or blue cheese dressing. Both are usually safe choices but read the labels. I remember during one of my rounds with Weight Watchers I learned to like mustard because we couldn't have ketchup. Stay away from honey mustards, though. I like the grainy-type mustards because I like the mouth feel. For more lunches, let's not forget leftovers! And soup! My dinners might look like this:

- Grass-fed (or regular) ground beef broiled with a slice of cheese (please no American or processed "cheese food"), a salad with olive oil and vinegar, steamed asparagus or string beans topped with slivered almonds that have been sautéed in a little butter. The family can add rolls for the burger and sweet potato fries (which you can have too at this point!).

- Chicken thighs (or a whole chicken) roasted with fresh garlic and white wine, salad with dressing (oil and vinegar, blue cheese or ranch) and broccoli or Brussels sprouts roasted with garlic and topped with crumbled bacon. The family can have a serving of rice or a baked potato (you, too, can have a baked potato but make it a medium-sized one). I make a roast chicken every Sunday at my daughter's house using plenty of garlic and lemon, and so far, no one has tired of it yet!

- Flank steak cut into strips and sautéed with three-colored bell peppers and sliced onions served with mashed or riced cauliflower. There need be no addition for the family other than if they would like tortillas to wrap the stir-fry. If you want to eliminate the wraps but want to serve a starch, you can make a very small potato dice and sauté with the meat and vegetables. If you blanch the potatoes after dicing and then add to the mixture, the starch (and thus sugar) will be reduced.

- Oven-roasted pork chops with shredded cabbage sautéed with butter, onions and a touch of apple cider vinegar.

Please note that no recipes are needed for any of these. They are family-friendly meals, and they travel well for lunch the next day. Please notice as well that I am not serving meals that deprive me, or the family, of good and delicious food. They do not take hours of prep, grocery shopping or cooking. Understand that if you have been relying heavily on processed foods to prepare meals, take-out or pasta-heavy meals, then yes, it will be an adjustment for everyone not just you. But if you have a family to feed, their health will improve too. When you shop and cook this way it is actually less expensive. Think of the dollars saved if you are cutting down on junk food (chips, cookies, snack food) or take-out, fast-food meals, processed foods (boxed and canned foods that you either use to prepare meals or serve on the side), breakfast junk (pop tarts, instant breakfasts, ready-made burritos or breakfast sandwiches, etc.) or your own snacking.

If your meals come from a family culture whose food heavily uses grains and legumes, it may be another adjustment. In this case you might need to offer more "sides" to your family but keep going back to your WHY (Chapter 19) and remind yourself over and over and over again about what is important to you. When I was preparing content for my course *Breaking Free From Diet Prison: The Roadmap to Low Carb and Keto Success*™ (miriamhatoum.com) I researched the cooking for several of these cultures. I was surprised at the volume of recipes that use no grains or grain products where you would expect them. These included Mexican, Dominican, Latino, Italian, Chinese and German recipes.

At this point in the game, you might need to sit down with your family and explain why you are doing this. Explain that you will do your best to continue finding meals that you all can enjoy as a family, but that you would appreciate it if they would support the way you are eating and trying to change your life. Ask that they do not tempt you, for fun or otherwise, with what is on their own plates. Put out a family challenge to find recipes that they would enjoy and that would fit into the new way you are eating. With little ones, make a challenge of asking what some of their favorite foods are and how you could make them healthier or what might be a good substitution. Make fun kid foods such as "ants on a log" – peanut butter on a celery stick topped with raisins. Even you can have that if you get a good healthy peanut or almond butter and use only two or three raisins. You are not asking your entire family to change, just to be supportive of you. Sometimes a side of spaghetti or a baked potato with plenty of toppings will hush the objections!

MINDFULNESS PRACTICE

At this step, maybe even more than when you gave up sugar, you might be missing your snacks of chips, pretzels and popcorn, or your sides of pasta and beans. Your mindfulness practice for this step is built upon Michelle May's "Am I Hungry" series. Stop and ask yourself, "What do I want? What do I need? What do I have?" Let's take this through to its conclusion:

I want popcorn. I want to crunch and have the hand-to-mouth feel.

I don't really need it. I am just scratching an itch or feeding a habit.

I will find something else to do.

IT ENDS HERE.

OR

I want popcorn. I want to crunch and have the hand-to-mouth experience.

I don't really need it. I am just scratching an itch or feeding a habit.

But I want it. What do I have? I have some vegetables that will give me crunch and satisfy the hand-to-mouth feel. OH HEAVENS. I don't want vegetables.

IT ENDS HERE.

OR

I want popcorn. I want to crunch and have the hand-to-mouth feel.

I don't really need it. I am just scratching an itch or feeding a habit.

But I want it. What do I have? I have some vegetables that will give me crunch and satisfy the hand-to-mouth feel.

I will have a few pickles or make a small bowl of carrots, celery and cucumber sticks.

IT'S OVER.

Whatever scenario plays out, the point is you have brought mindfulness to it. That alone sometimes is enough to stop the chatter in its tracks. If you are hungry EAT. Putting a pause between thinking of the food and reaching for the food is sometimes enough to realize you are not hungry and you are thinking about food out of habit.

Oh, and p.s. YOU DON'T NEED BREAD! Have you figured that out already?

GOOD TO KNOW...

In addition to the sheer carbohydrate content of grains and legumes there are other reasons why I suggest limiting or eliminating them on low carb and keto eating plans. When eaten as a staple food, they simply crowd out more nutritious foods like animal products. They contain phytic acid and lectins which can interfere with absorption of nutrition and in some cases, be responsible for inflammation. Combined with the phytic acid and lack of fats in the grains and legumes themselves, this can lead to possible nutritional deficiency. Time-consuming preparations such as soaking, sprouting, and fermenting can mitigate some problems, but they are still high in carbohydrates. If you must eat them, do so sparingly and only occasionally.

Chapter Five

Step 3: Learn About and Lower Your Carbs

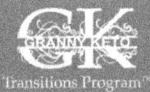

Step 3

Limited carbohydrates

This step is where you become aware of the carbohydrate counts of fruits, vegetables, dairy, nuts, grains and legumes. I wrestled with having this as Step 1, but in that step I did not want you to be hampered with eliminating foods and worrying about the carbohydrate count of what you did decide to eat. It was important first to be comfortable with starting to change your eating lifestyle before getting into the nitty-gritty of counting carbohydrates.

My hope is that you will be able to shift your eating style to a more conservative and healthy way of consuming carbohydrates. The carbohydrate count in the Standard American Diet (often referred to as SAD) can be, conservatively, 400 to 500 or more carbohydrates per day even if you are not overeating or bingeing. Jimmy Moore, a pioneer in this field, said that when he finally counted his daily carbohydrate intake, he realized that he was consuming thousands of carbohydrates with all the soda he was drinking and snacks he was eating! These carbohydrates add up – one meal will usually have 100 or more! Take a moderate, typical breakfast:

8 oz juice: 27 carbs

1 cup multi-grain cheerios: 24 carbs

Small, sliced banana: 24 carbs

1 cup 2% milk: 12 carbs

Coffee with 2 TBS creamer: 10 carbs.

*Total: 95 carbs.

Want to add a Starbucks® or Dunkin Donuts® coffee drink to that on the way to work? Depending upon whether you use a flavoring and/or sugar, it can add up to another 40 carbs for a small one. ONE multi-grain bagel – nothing even on it: 63 carbs! Okay forget the Starbucks coffee drink and maybe the bagel.

What are things you might pick up as a snack or add to your meal during the day? Think you are "good" to get just a snack bag of BAKED Lays® potato chips? Add 23 carbs right there for only fifteen chips – and that is probably only half a snack bag. Think a handful of grapes (about one cup) is better? Well maybe – that's only 29 carbs.

Lunch? Boy, you're being good here – you brought one of these Lean Cuisines to heat up at work. Examples:

Sesame Chicken: 51 carb

Glazed Turkey Tenderloins: 44 carbs

Lasagna with Meat Sauce: 45 carbs

Parmesan Crusted Fish: 42 carbs.

AND let me add, as a former Lean Cuisine and Weight Watchers frozen-meal sort of gal – you are STARVING within an hour so let's add fruit, salad, maybe popcorn or pretzels, etc. Haven't switched to diet soda to go with that Lean Cuisine? A can of Coke is 40 carbs. You get the point here – by the time your day is done with three meals and two to three snacks, you are easily looking at 400 to 500 carbs or more. I spared you going through a dinner menu that might include a baked potato, or pasta, bread, a casserole that might have breading, etc. – but you get the point from what goes on at breakfast and lunch.

Okay! Enough! So, what can you do? Low carb eating might be a great step for you to land on and find success. If you plan to stay at low carb (Step 3) for a while, there are many ways to do it. Usually, 30 to 50 carbohydrate grams of carbohydrates per meal is what you will be comfortable eating. If you are staying at this step, try to eat under 150 carbohydrates a day for a week or two and then check your weight. If your goal is weight loss on low carb and it is not happening for you, cut back a little further. This is a good step to acquaint yourself with cutting back if your goal is to become fully keto where you probably will be starting with 20 carbohydrates for the day. If you start with 30 to 40 carbs per meal (which is still considered low carb) practice cutting back further if your plan is to go all the way to keto. If you have already gone through TRANSITIONS STEPS 1 and 2, you are no longer eating sugar, baked goods, grains or any grain product, and legumes. It will also likely mean that you are eating very few packaged and processed foods. You are almost there! If you want to accelerate weight loss you can further cut back on starchy vegetables and fruit (TRANSITIONS STEPS 4 and 5). Eating in a low carb way has a lot of leeway. Again, that is a personal decision to be dictated by your goals (reducing inflammation, losing weight, working your way towards keto, etc.).

Don't worry about following a particular low carb diet (*Living Low Carb* by Jonny Bowden presents 23 popular ones – all a little different in how many carbs are allowed in a day or how to approach the diet). DANCING WITH LOW CARB AND KETO (CHAPTER 13) is appropriate with both low carb and keto, and in that chapter, I give you examples of dancing with both. The premise is, that once you have taken the time to learn carbohydrate counts of various foods you can start to trust yourself to have the knowledge about what to eat and in what quantities. If you have worked your way through Steps 1 and 2, you have already reduced some of the big offenders of carbohydrates (sugars, grains, legumes) but you still have to learn about the carbohydrates in starchy vegetables:

potatoes (white and sweet), corn (corn is a grain but is also sometimes considered a vegetable; you may not have given it up in Transitions Step 2), peas, parsnips, etc. You will also become aware of sugar vegetables such as beets, carrots, sweet bell peppers and tomatoes (technically a fruit but considered a vegetable). All vegetables are carbohydrates. Be aware of your portion sizes, even if it is broccoli, asparagus or zucchini. Leafy greens are the least offenders, and, in any case, it would be to your advantage to have a large leafy salad or leafy-green shake daily – just watch your dressings on the salads and add little to no fruit to your shakes.

It is possible (and preferred) to eat in a low carb way that does not require you to count carbohydrates. This is truly breaking free from diet prison. If you limit your fruit intake to one or two per day and limit a carb-heavy food (i.e., rice, potatoes, etc.) to once or twice a day and a small dessert no more than once or twice a week, you will find your way to this food freedom. You can find food freedom with limitation and not necessarily elimination.

However, it does all start with awareness. If you want to get a more detailed lay of the land, skip ahead to Chapter 9, Understanding Keto, for a discussion about net carbs, total carbs and Granny Keto's hybrid way of counting carbs. If you want to start out by tracking and counting carbohydrates, explore which way you might like to do it. Try it one way for a week or two. If you are not successful with your weight loss, try a different way or lower the carbohydrate count you are allowing yourself. My hope for you is that once you are familiar with high carbohydrate foods you will be able to eat in a way where this sort of tracking is no longer necessary.

Whether to count total carbohydrates or net carbohydrates is based on whether or not your body has an insulin response to fiber. This is also a decision you have to make on your own. You will make it based on blood glucose readings, if you are taking them, after you have eaten certain foods. Without blood glucose readings you can base the decision on the way you feel after eating a certain food. If your weight loss has stalled, that is another way to make the decision. If you have started counting net carbs (which is subtracting fiber and sugar alcohols) you may want to move to counting total carbs (which is the full carbohydrate count of a food, not subtracting anything). Again, please read Chapter 9 to help you with this decision.

Your ultimate goal is to get out of the diet prison of weighing, measuring and tracking your foods. At the start of this process, I do suggest that you write things down or at least look up the various foods that you think might be high in carbohydrates (maybe even just one or two days a week) so that you build an awareness of what you are eating. Eventually you will be able to make decisions that usually are spot on with regard to portion sizes and carbohydrate counts. Coaching my clients to eat from the Yes/No list in Chapter 9 but allowing them to have a conservative amount of carbohydrate sources (bread, rice, potatoes, etc.), has proven quite successful. However, in order to find food freedom, you must also do the mindfulness practices given to you throughout these chapters. Getting familiar with your "hunger scale" is particularly important. I love the expression about "picking your hard." It might be a little difficult at the beginning to do your mindfulness practices, but it will save you from years of being in diet prison. Pick your hard.

FRUIT

Don't have your head in the sand about fruit. While you are following a low carb eating style, you can have fruit. However, I think the biggest downfall of some of the popular diets is that fruit is unlimited. A cup of grapes is 29 carbohydrates, and half a medium cantaloupe is 23 carbohydrates. You might say – who eats a half a cantaloupe? If you are my age – in your 60s, surely you remember putting cottage cheese in the well of half a cantaloupe! A fresh Bartlett pear is 25 carbohydrates and a small banana in our breakfast example is 24 carbohydrates. There are, of course, many fruits with fewer carbohydrates, but I want you to build an awareness and a mindfulness when you reach for fruit. The reason fruits are not allowed on keto (if you are heading that way you might as well have the information now) is because they are made up of fructose, sucrose and glucose. Fructose, specifically, puts a heavy burden on the liver. No cell in the body can directly use fructose so it goes directly to the liver and can be responsible for problems you may be having with losing weight, and particularly belly fat. You should limit your fruits to very low carbohydrate ones (the lower carb count indicates less sugar) and limit the amount you eat in a day to no more than one or two. Forget the gigantic fruit salads you think are so wonderful! When you get to keto you will be eating only berries and limited lemon and lime juices of one to two tablespoons for flavoring.

DAIRY AND EGGS

When you start to eat a low carb lifestyle, please be aware of carbohydrates in dairy products and eggs. The carbohydrates in dairy can add up during the course of the day. Please do not use fake powdered or liquid creamers in your coffee. Aside from all the chemicals and junk in these creamers, just one tablespoon (sugar-free) can be upwards of five carbohydrates or more. And really – do you only use ONE tablespoon? Half & half or light cream will be better; heavy cream will be best! We are not watching fat in this, or any step.

Pay particular attention to yogurt. "Light" yogurts can run 20 or more carbohydrates, and regular yogurt with fruit and flavorings can carry a price tag of 40 or more carbohydrates. Even if you go directly to plain yogurt, you can be looking at 15 or more carbohydrates per 8 ounces. Check your brands carefully. At this point, even with keto, it is okay to count only half of the carbohydrates present in plain full-fat yogurt. This is because yogurt products are labeled with their properties prior to the conversion of the milk to yogurt. Enzymes present in the process will convert the lactose to lactic acid. Remember, this is only for plain full-fat yogurt.

Please stay away from processed cheese "foods" and anything flavored. It is fine to consume cheese but be aware that the carbohydrates add up. I am not putting eggs in here to keep you away from them (they truly are a perfect food) but I want to bring your attention to the fact that even a food we consider to be protein can also have carbohydrates! Egg substitutes have more carbohydrates and less protein than real eggs. EAT REAL EGGS AND EAT THE YOLKS!

SEEDS AND NUTS

Feel free to have nuts at this level, but I strongly urge you not to grab a handful of any of them. Nuts and seeds, probably more than anything else, will stall your weight loss. This is not because inherently there is anything wrong with nuts. Many nuts provide a great way to find something filling that has healthy fat and protein, but they all have carbohydrates. If you aren't careful, you will be consuming ten or more carbohydrates in a tiny handful (tiny = if you had your four-year-old grandson take them out of the package for you). Nut butters are also okay, but again, measure! If you are careful about taking small portions of nuts or seeds (two tablespoons to one quarter of a cup, at most) you will also not be in danger of too much fat or protein. But still, even with watching yourself, have nuts and seeds be the first things you look at if you are in a serious stall.

OTHER FOODS TO WATCH FOR

In GRANNY KETO TRANSITIONS PROGRAM™ STEPS 1 and 2, we work on eliminating sugar, baked goods, grains, and legumes. At Transitions Step 3 you may have these items (if it is not your intention to go to keto) but do so cautiously. Be aware that "whole grain" or "light" bread products, crackers, and cereals are not any better for you than anything else that has been packaged. If you eventually hit a point where you are, or desire to be, fully keto, and start looking at Facebook pages and keto websites, you will see the term: "If it fits your macros" (discussed in the Appendix). Basically, what this means is that if you decide to eat 20 total carbs, you can eat anything as long as it doesn't come to more than 20 total carbs. Many low carb diets subscribe to this approach allowing these foods that we have limited or eliminated in Steps 1 and 2. I do not subscribe to "if it fits your macros" if you follow keto. It is not just the carb count that makes a difference in your weight loss and health. Grains cause inflammation in your gut and body. Fructose hits your liver hard and greatly contributes to conditions such as insulin resistance and type 2 diabetes. When you are eating so few carbohydrates on keto, or any level of low carb, make them count. Eat fresh vegetables, dairy, eggs, etc. Don't waste them on things like ketchup, "light" bread and pasta.

You can learn to make the best choices within your low carb limits and allowances even if you do not have a book or the Internet available when you sit down at a meal or go grocery shopping. You are an intelligent human being and for sure you know that at a party, an appetizer of crudités, cheese, olives and a few crackers is a lower carb choice than chips, pretzels and savory party breads.

At a lunch restaurant, a Cobb salad topped with deli meats, eggs, bacon and blue cheese crumbles is a better choice than a burger with the bun with sides of onion rings and French fries. These are "extreme" examples and sometimes the differences in choices may not be as glaring. But you will eventually come to trust your knowledge and be able to engage in the practice of "Good-Better-Best" which is just what it implies. Look at your choices and pick something that is not outrageously out of your carbohydrate parameters (GOOD). Can you tweak it by leaving off the bread or saying no to croutons and the side of potatoes (BETTER)? Can you go further and order something that you absolutely know will fit your parameters such as steak or chicken (no breading), salad (no croutons), a green vegetable and fruit for dessert (BEST)?

MINDFULNESS PRACTICE

This step's mindfulness practice calls for you to pay attention to what you are eating and how the food or quantity of food makes you feel. Think about how you might adjust the meal the next time you eat these foods, if you were not satisfied by the meal, if you didn't feel well, if it made you sleepy or you found you were hungry soon after. Equally important is to notice if the meal or individual food made you feel good (not just the lack of not feeling well). Did the meal give you energy? Did it satisfy you for several hours?

Let's use potatoes for an example. As you are cutting down sugars and foods that turn into glucose in your body, you might find that you are becoming sensitive to heavier carbohydrates. A baked potato that never bothered you now feels heavy in your stomach. All vegetables are carbohydrates, but a potato will feel different in your body than a salad would. You might find that these starchier and heavier carbohydrate foods make you sleepy, make you hungry sooner or even unsettle your stomach.

Start to pay attention to those things. It will help you make smarter choices so that you use your carbohydrates more wisely. It will also help you immensely if your goal is to be fully keto. A well-formulated keto diet has a lot to do with what foods you are eating and in what quantities they satisfy you. You will start tuning into hunger and satiety signals. If you want to move away from weighing and measuring, listen to your body to know that you have picked the right foods and quantities for satiety. This mindfulness practice is an important step to help you get – and stay – out of diet prison.

GOOD TO KNOW...

What are carbohydrates? Carbohydrates are sugars and starches that the body breaks down into glucose (a simple sugar that the body can use to feed its cells). Cellulose and fiber are also carbohydrates but are unlikely to turn into sugar in your body, as they pass, undigested, through the digestive system. However, some people are sensitive to them and that is why they do not subtract them from their carbohydrate totals. The difference between the different carbohydrates lies in the number of sugar molecules they contain. Simple carbs, also known as simple sugars, contain one or two sugar molecules. Foods known as complex carbs have three or more sugar molecules. So no, a carrot doesn't turn into chocolate cake when it hits your bloodstream, but it is broken down into simple glucose the way a piece of cake would break down.

Chapter Six
Step 4: Moderate Protein and No Fruit Except Berries

(For Low Carb you will be limiting fruits, not eliminating them.)

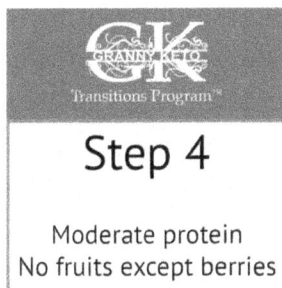

Step 4

Moderate protein
No fruits except berries

The information in this step is valuable whether you are eating low carb or will be following the keto path. It will help you with your decisions about fruit and protein as you aim for lower carbohydrate intake and higher protein consumption. It is important to realize that our habit of reaching for fruit as a snack might not be the best option for us. It is also essential to understand the importance of protein.

Fruit

I would have started keto six months sooner had I not heard "No fruit except for berries." I said, "No way am I ever giving up fruit. Are they crazy?" But then I started learning more, allowed myself to be more open-minded and accepted the truth.

There are a few issues with fruit. Let's just start with the pure sugar and carbohydrate content of fruits. If you are going to be fully keto you will be restricting your carbohydrates. Here are examples of the carbohydrates in some fruits, with the counts varying by size.

- Peach (12)
- Orange (16)
- Apple (25)
- Pear (25)
- Banana (24)

Berries, by contrast, in moderation (about ½ cup) not only have much less sugar but their glycemic load is also low, meaning they will very slowly, if at all, raise a person's blood glucose level. The glycemic load measures the amount of carbohydrates in a serving of food. The glycemic index measures how rapidly a carbohydrate is released as glucose (sugar) into the blood.

In terms of how many carbohydrates you ingest and how quickly those carbohydrates hit your system, fruit is a poor nutritional choice. What about vitamins and nutrients, you ask? You will get what you need from vegetables and animal products. There are no essential nutrients in fruit that outweigh the harm because of the amount of sugar in them. The biggest fallacy is that you need oranges and other citrus foods to get Vitamin C. In fact, bell peppers, chili peppers, kale, broccoli, cauliflower and Brussels sprouts are just some vegetables that will deliver a good punch of this vitamin. In essence, there are no essential nutrients and vitamins that you will miss by eliminating or limiting fruit.

However, there is a more serious concern with fruit that goes beyond counting carbohydrates. Fructose, one of the sugars in fruit, cannot be used by your cells for energy. Fructose goes directly to the liver to be metabolized. It is ultimately one of the major causes of non-alcoholic fatty liver disease which is linked to early death, diabetes and heart disease. Fruit also makes you more insulin resistant, raises your triglycerides, increases inflammation and has a terrible effect on your cholesterol. More and more studies are being done on this. There are already many animal studies, but the link is so strong and interesting that more human studies are also being conducted. These studies include learning about the difference between fructose in fruits, HFCS (high-fructose corn syrup) and combinations of fructose and glucose. From where things stand now, many researchers consider fructose to be a liver toxin because of the work the liver has to do to metabolize it.

When I listened to *Why We Get Fat and What to Do About It* by Gary Taubes, everything finally fell into place for me, and I immediately gave up fruit and started keto. It was over a year before I even ate a berry! I finally understood why I never lost a pound even though I faithfully followed a Paleo lifestyle for years. It was all the sugar in the unlimited fruits I was eating along with other allowed elements of Paleo, including no limit on root vegetables, nuts, honey, etc. The fruit-to-insulin connection and then what insulin is responsible for, opened my eyes and enabled me to accept keto.

For this step, if you have decided to do keto, I ask that you cut out fruit. I would further suggest that you not have berries at this point in your transition to keto, but if you must, please limit them to ½ cup per day. If you are doing keto, you may want to do some investigation. For instance, blueberries are higher in sugar than other berries so try to go with raspberries, strawberries or blackberries.

If you are eating low carb, you may continue to eat fruits but please limit them to one or two servings a day. It is also important to note (for the low carb eaters) that dried fruits and tropical fruits have a high concentration of sugar, and thus would be very high carbohydrate choices. The carbohydrates and fructose do not concern me if you limit them, but they may keep sugar cravings alive, and if you are still battling the sugar demon even after TRANSITIONS STEPS 1 and 2, it might work in your favor to eliminate all fruits and berries for a while. You can always add them back once you no longer have cravings that take you off course.

Keto allows the juice of fresh lemons and limes because the sugar/carbohydrate count is very low. However – and not that anyone would – please don't drink a glass of pure lemon or lime juice! A couple of tablespoons of these juices throughout the day to flavor your foods and beverages are okay. Again, if you are taking the low carb path in your journey, there is no "rule" to eliminate fruit but keep your fruit intake to those with lower carbohydrate counts such as grapefruits and melons.

Learn which are the high-sugar fruits (grapes, bananas, dried fruits, etc.) and do your best to stay away from them. And, just as with keto, have the only juices you use be for flavoring, not drinking.

If you are doing keto and you are concerned about your reliance on fruit, don't have fruit for a day or two. Then a week. Then before you know it, you won't miss it at all. I remember when I started, I told my friend, "I can't imagine never eating another piece of watermelon for the rest of my life." The rest of your life is a long time. Don't look at that now. If you have type 2 diabetes, insulin resistance or any other form of metabolic disorder, these can almost always be healed with a well-formulated keto diet. There might come a time when you can have a piece of fresh fruit and not have your insulin and blood sugars go all wonky. More importantly, there will be a time, once you are not only physically healed but emotionally healed as well, when you can have a piece of fruit and not have the craving monster plague you. But for right now, for just this day in front of you, don't reach for that piece of fruit. Trust me on this, please. I went through my first three summers of keto without a piece of watermelon and I survived. The first summer I enjoyed some watermelon and I did not feel the need to binge on an entire serving plate of watermelon and other fruits. When I measured my blood glucose in the evening it was all good which indicated that my insulin resistance was healing! Yours will too.

Are you used to taking a piece of fruit for a snack? That was the hardest for me, even more than giving up those fruit salads and plates of fresh watermelon. Once you start working on Step 5 (high fat) you most likely will not have the urge to snack anymore, at least not because of hunger (eating from boredom or habit is another issue!). Here are some ideas for snacks:

- Salami & cheese, or just a piece of string or hard cheese
- Celery and cream cheese or unsweetened nut butter
- Broth with butter – don't laugh – sometimes I will have that when I "need" a snack. Often, I have that and find myself so full and satisfied, I don't even want my next meal!
- Nuts
- Kale or spinach smoothie (no fruit!)
- Roast beef rollup
- Hard boiled eggs

You can see that there is plenty to reach for and it doesn't have to be an apple or banana! As you cut out fruit your need to snack on it will lessen.

PROTEIN

MODERATE – BUT DO NOT FEAR – YOUR PROTEIN INTAKE. If your target here is to be fully keto, understand that you are not going to be eating unlimited amounts of protein. However, you should not be worried about eating too much. As a matter of fact, at the time of publication of this book, no organization has established a firm upper limit on what might constitute too much protein in a person's diet. Also, in a healthy individual, the body can safely rid itself of unneeded protein. Protein is an essential nutrient and the building blocks of cells and muscles. It is essential for brain function and other functions, such as healing cuts and wounds. The body "recycles" much of its protein and you do not need to consume large quantities to be healthy.

If you are interested in keto, you may have heard of gluconeogenesis, where the liver can convert amino acids (from protein) into glucose. In this case the liver may produce a little too much glucose, which could impact insulin. However, gluconeogenesis is usually not a supply-driven process. It is mostly a demand-driven process, meaning that it doesn't automatically happen if you eat a lot of protein. It happens if and when your body needs glucose. The issue of the liver converting protein into excessive glucose tends to happen more in people with very severe insulin resistance or difficult-to-control diabetes.

Another thing to consider if you tend to eat a lot of protein is that protein contains a lot of phosphorus which is a stimulant. You will find you might not sleep well after a heavy protein dinner!

The term "grams of protein" means the number of grams of protein that is in a food, not the weight of the food in grams. For example, three ounces of ground chuck, cooked, weighs 85 grams and contains 22 grams of protein. The same three ounces (85g) of cooked bacon, contains 9 grams of protein. This is a question that comes up frequently when people are new to keto. Not to worry – just make sure you are measuring the correct thing! To measure how much protein you "should" be eating, there are various calculations and formulas based on height, body mass, or other factors such as BMR (Basal Metabolic Rate) and TDEE (Total Daily Energy Expenditure). However, human beings are not machines, and calculators should not rule your life. Once you are adept at using the Mindfulness Practice in this step (Your Hunger Scale), you will become aware of the amount of protein that is comfortable for your body.

When you are beginning keto or low carb eating, the only metric you have to pay attention to is your carbohydrate count. If you follow keto you will see a lot of references to your "macros" (how many grams you are allowed of each category: carbohydrates, protein, and fat). I do want you to be informed about what you are reading. However, I do not agree with the extremely low protein allotment that most keto sites will give you. One such calculation for keto-protein allotment is 45.5 grams per 5' of height, then every inch over five feet, multiply by 2.3 and add it to 45.5. There are other formulas that may include body mass, BMR, and TDEE. If you are young, an athlete, and not metabolically challenged in any way, you certainly can have more than whatever that calculation comes out to be. If you are not losing weight, not getting into ketosis (explained in Chapter 9, but "low carbers" do not have to be concerned with the term), have conditions such as non-alcoholic fatty liver disease (NAFLD), are severely insulin resistant, have type 2 diabetes, etc., you may want to work within that calculated number and pay close attention to the "incidental" protein that I talk about below.

The following is an example of a more realistic (and backed by research) protein calculation if you are more comfortable working with numbers right now. It is 1.2 to 1.7 grams per kilogram of "reference" body weight. The reference weight is not your goal weight necessarily, but what is an average weight for your height. For instance, I am 5'4" and my "reference" body weight is approximately 140 pounds (64 kg). I got this by using a standard BMI chart, looking up my height and picking the number that falls at the high end of a "normal" BMI, which is 24. (We can split hairs here: normal is up to 24.9 but then the math gets too hard!) My protein allowance falls between 76.8 to 108.8 grams of consumed protein (not grams of weight).

What does this look like for meals? When you start out, you will probably be eating three meals a day. I recommend STRONGLY that you limit yourself to three adequate meals that cut out any need for snacking. Start with that and arrange your protein grams accordingly. The best way to approach this is to split your protein fairly evenly between these three meals which comes out to about 30 grams of protein per meal. This is main-course protein. There is also "incidental" protein in vegetables, coffee cream, cheese, nuts and seeds. When I started keto, I paid no attention to limiting protein. As I stopped losing weight, it was the first thing that my coach and I looked at. I cut slightly back on protein, mostly paying more attention to the "incidentals" rather than cutting back on my main meal proteins.

Use your mindfulness practices to pay attention to what you eat and learn protein counts of food. At the beginning of my journey when I did count "macros" (carbohydrate, protein and fat), just to get things in line, I did look things up and I was so surprised to find that fish and shellfish and other lean protein pack a lot of protein into each serving size. As long as you are eating good quality protein, don't worry too much about that. It is unlikely that a woman is going to overeat protein (in fact, most women are not getting enough!) and you don't have to run back and forth to your food scale to shave off an ounce of something. You need to make this a lifestyle and not a diet. As with carbohydrates, once you have an awareness of what you are eating you can let go of the tracking and break free from diet prison.

Eat good quality protein and pay attention to your hunger signals. If you are still afraid of protein after all you have read on social media and want to avoid overeating, one doctor (Robert Cywes) has coined the term *sequential eating*. Some people, including myself, call it "putting in a speed bump." Take what you feel is an adequate portion of food and divide it onto two plates. Put the plate in front of you that you are going to eat and put the other plate either in the middle of the table or on a kitchen counter. Finish what is in front of you, then see if you want the rest. This is a great mindfulness practice to use. Do not take 3 ounces of protein (the standard "deck-of-cards" or "palm-of-your-hand" sized portion) and divide that. Take something substantially more to start so that half is at least 3 ounces. If you are still hungry and want to eat more, EAT MORE!!! Choose protein sources where the fat is part of the protein such as chicken thighs with the skin, egg yolks (not just the whites) or a steak that is marbled or has the fat layer around it, like a good ribeye. These choices will automatically align protein and fat recommendations and will keep you full longer on less food!

This step of protein awareness is NOT the final step in becoming fully keto. The final TRANSITIONS step (STEP 5) will be to learn to eat higher fat. Once you are doing that, and if you have already started a practice of eating enough protein, you will find it much easier to find a comfortable protein intake amount while following a keto diet. Don't make yourself crazy with macros but instead, begin to listen to your body. When you get to DANCING WITH LOW CARB AND KETO (CHAPTER 13) you will find your sweet spot with protein. Just a little more than some might recommend for keto might make you feel better (energy-wise and digestion-wise) and might make the difference between being successful or not.

Remember these two concepts when choosing how much protein to eat: We are not machines and must, instead, eat according to what makes us feel best. For some it might be a little more protein and a little less fat than a standard keto macro calculation would have you eating. DO NOT FEAR protein. Gluconeogenesis is a demand-driven process and not a supply-driven process.

MINDFULNESS PRACTICE

This step's mindfulness practice is a big one and is explored more fully in PART 4 — MAKING LOW CARB AND KETO A LIFESTYLE. Pay attention to your own personal hunger scale. Unless this is your very first time following a nutritional program, I am sure you have heard of the hunger and fullness scale. This is the one I like to use: Famished is a 1 and stuffed is a 10.

1. Ravenous and famished. You are starving, feeling faint or shaky.

2. Really hungry. You may be preoccupied with food.

   1–2: **TRY NOT TO ALLOW YOURSELF TO GET HERE**: You will make poor food choices and eat too fast.

3. Hungry. Ready for a meal but you don't feel like you need to stop everything and eat.

4. Hungry. You could put off eating a bit longer. Distraction will take your mind off food, but not for long.

   3–4: **THIS IS A GOOD PLACE TO EAT**: You will be able to make good food choices and not wolf down your food.

5. Neutral. If you are eating, you could stop here. Also, if you are not eating, your mind really doesn't go to food. You haven't hit 3 or 4 yet.

6. Satisfied. A little more might make you full, but you could finish what you are eating and not be stuffed.

    5–6: THIS IS A GOOD PLACE TO STOP EATING: You have enjoyed your meal and can easily walk away from anything that is left. You will stop thinking about food or you might notice about 20 minutes after finishing that you are comfortably full.

7. Full. You might start to feel a little uncomfortable and wish you didn't have those last few morsels.

8. Very Full. At this point you are definitely feeling uncomfortable, and definitely wishing you hadn't continued eating.

    7–8: STOP – REALLY: You might find that you are determined to also have a dessert with a meal. I'm telling you now: You'll be sorry. Please don't!

9. Overfull, stuffed, uncomfortable, bloated, stomachache.

10. Absolutely stuffed. You are not only uncomfortable, but you may be nauseous, sweating, need to sleep, and painfully full.

    9–10: FORGIVE YOURSELF. Then, if you can, get up and walk around. Don't make it worse by beating yourself up and punishing yourself by eating even more. If you find yourself here often then it is time to talk with a counselor or do some serious thought work and introspection. You are getting here not because the food tastes too good to stop. There are other, deeper issues, and I implore you to work on figuring them out.

Use these weeks on TRANSITIONS STEP 4 to get familiar with – and honor – your hunger scale. The more in tune you are to the cues, the more you are likely to be successful not only with "Dancing" (CHAPTER 13) but also developing and recognizing your own level of satiety.

One last word with regard to 7 to 10 of this scale: do not throw out the baby with the bathwater. This means that you could be going along fairly well. Then you get invited to a steakhouse where you order the 16 oz. prime rib and eat ALL of it (come on, you know you can!). I would have suggested cutting it in half immediately and boxing it up to take home for another meal. But you keep picking away at it until it is all gone in one sitting. Overeating is not a moral issue. Do not judge yourself. You ate a delicious piece of meat. I hope you enjoyed it! Don't eat less tomorrow or give up altogether. Just try to do better the next day or the next meal and be a little more mindful and a lot more careful! I tell myself – OFTEN – "This way of eating is a way of life. It is not a religion." Things happen. You make mistakes. You make poor decisions. You make foolish decisions. To whom does that not happen – sometimes on a regular basis? Forgive yourself. Actually, there is nothing to forgive. Move on. In the next step we will be saying: **KETO ON!!!!**

GOOD TO KNOW...

This is from Harvard Publishing: The entry of fructose into the liver kicks off a series of complex chemical transformations. One remarkable change is that the liver uses fructose, a carbohydrate, to create fat. This process is called lipogenesis. Give the liver enough fructose, and tiny fat droplets begin to accumulate in liver cells. This buildup is called non-alcoholic fatty liver disease, because it looks just like what happens in the livers of people who drink too much alcohol. Virtually unknown before 1980, non-alcoholic fatty liver disease now affects up to 30% of adults in the United States and other developed countries, and between 70% and 90% of those who are obese or who have diabetes.

Chapter Seven

Step 5: Eat Higher Fat and Eliminate Starchy Vegetables

(For Low Carb you will be limiting, not eliminating, starchy vegetables.)

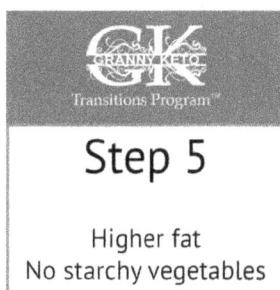

Step 5

Higher fat
No starchy vegetables

You have made it to the last Transitions step before going on to being fully keto if that is where you are headed. At this step you will probably be eating more fat than you ever have before. By this time in the program, it is helpful if you are choosing fatty proteins: brisket, corned beef, 80/20 ground beef (80% lean with 20% fat), salmon, chicken thighs and legs – with skin, and deli cuts such as salami. Hopefully you are no longer cutting the fat off steaks. The keto rule is to eat fat to satiety, but it may still be difficult for you to know what satiety is (do the hunger scale work in Chapters 6 and 12!). Granted, it is one of the harder things to learn about your own body. When you have no sense of what your body is telling you, it may be helpful to pay attention to your fat macros at first even though ultimately you will not be tracking. Learn to connect what you have eaten with how you are feeling.

The Calories-In-Calories-Out (CICO) hypothesis no longer holds water at this point because now we are dealing with the true source of weight gain and stubborn fat loss: hormones, and specifically INSULIN. Insulin is the fat-storage hormone and we have been reducing it all through the Transitions process. At this step you will further reduce insulin by eliminating or limiting starchy and root vegetables. Up to now the starchy vegetables may have filled your plate instead of sugars and grains. But now, without them, how do you fill your plate so that you are satisfied?

Fat

Fat is the only nutrient that generates little to no insulin response. That's exactly what we want. It has nothing to do with calories. Besides, if you are keeping your carbohydrates low and your protein adequate, no matter how you add fat to your day, it most likely will not bring you to excessive calories. Just in case you don't believe me and need further convincing on this, see these calculations:

- 20 total carbohydrates @ 4 calories per gram = 80 calories

- 100 grams of protein @ 4 calories per gram = 400 calories

- 100 grams of fat @ 9 calories per gram = 900 calories

This is a total of 1380 calories, enough to lose weight. Actually 1380 calories might be too low for most people to be comfortable. Do not eat more carbohydrates. Instead "play" with fat and then protein. As you eat more fat you remain fuller longer so there is no need for snacks. You may find yourself naturally moving to one or two meals a day instead of three. Do not concern yourself with calories. Do pay attention to your carbohydrates. The 1:1 ratio above (fat to protein, or grams of fat equaling grams of protein) is actually very low. Move it along to 1.5:1 (1 ½ grams of fat for every gram of protein). With 20g carbs, 100g protein and 150g fat you will still be eating a reasonable amount of food to lose weight – but ONLY if you keep your carbs in the vicinity of 20! Also remember that a gram is the amount of nutrient in the food, not the weight of the food. The goal of this program is to unlock the doors to diet prison. Low carbohydrate count, even with higher protein and fat will do that for you!

If you are coming from a very low-fat diet, do not have a gallbladder or have gallbladder issues, add your fats slowly. However, if you have already started picking the fattier proteins as suggested in Step 4, you will have already titrated to adequate fat, most likely without any negative consequence. Keto can be safe with no gallbladder. I had mine removed 35 years ago! I did, however, have to cut back on going to a full 2:1 fat-to-protein ratio at the beginning and build up to that. It took maybe a week or two before I no longer felt uncomfortable from the fat. I also took digestive enzymes to help with the breaking down of fat until my body adjusted to the higher intake of fat.

Because my children (now in their 30 and 40s) were raised by a fat-phobic mother, they grew up with boneless and skinless chicken breasts, 97% lean ground beef, white fish like cod and NEVER butter on vegetables! While it was very easy for me to switch to high fat (because I grew up in a chicken-fat sort of household), they cannot bring themselves to add fat to anything or eat the fat on meat. If you find yourself in that camp, especially with eating fattier meats, poultry and fish, you can add fat to your diet by easier means. Hardly anyone has trouble with butter, once given the permission to eat it! Take those boneless skinless chicken breasts and stuff them with high fat cheese and ham or bacon and bake or fry them basting in butter and then pour a lovely cream sauce (heavy cream, butter and lots of Parmesan cheese) over them. For kosher or halal households: You do NOT have to eat bacon, other pork products or dairy with meat. There are plenty of other ways to get your fats in while you are eating your protein.

The macro count on fat can be 1:1 (fat to protein) up to 2 (or more):1 (fat to protein) or somewhere in between. For me, if I am eating 100 grams of protein, I feel best if I am eating around 150 grams of fat. Even on the days I used to track, my fat and protein intake would be a little more or a little less than what I set out for it to be. I pay attention to whether I have enough fat and protein to feel satisfied, not whether I have had too many or too few grams (or calories).

Making fried eggs for breakfast? Use lots of butter. Having salad for lunch? Add olives, cheese and/or salami and top it with plenty of oil or a good blue cheese or ranch dressing. As long as you have enough carbohydrates and protein left for the remainder of your day, a handful of nuts can also add great fats.

The MYTH (known as the Diet-Heart hypothesis) is that fats (especially saturated fats) are bad for you. As a matter of fact, they serve very important functions such as building cell walls and aiding in mineral absorption and conversion of vitamins and minerals into forms that your body can use. For instance, the fat-soluble vitamins A, D, E, K are called fat soluble for a reason! If you eat low-fat or no-fat, you don't get the full nutrients in these vitamins.

Please do your best to stay away from polyunsaturated fats. Polyunsaturated fatty acids (PUFAs) can be dangerous for several reasons. Because of their structure, they are chemically unstable and susceptible to damage from heat, light and oxygen, causing them to oxidize thus causing high levels of inflammation in our bodies. These are mostly the industrial oils such as corn oil, peanut oil, "vegetable" oil, soybean oil and canola oil. Although many fats have naturally occurring PUFAs, they will not be identified as the main source of fatty acids. Bacon is 11% PUFA but identified as a saturated fat. There is no need to include excess PUFAs in your diet intentionally by using corn oil for frying, for instance. For more information on essential PUFAs such as omega-3 and omega-6 fatty acids, see my website.

Also stay away from trans fats that are found in many foods including fried foods like doughnuts and baked goods, including cakes, pie crusts, biscuits, frozen pizza, cookies, crackers, stick margarines and other spreads, the totally "plastic" whipped toppings, Crisco, and hundreds of processed food products. These are the fats that contribute to heart disease, obesity, diabetes, inflammation, IBS and other diseases. You can determine the amount of trans fats in a particular packaged food by looking at the nutrition panel. Do not be fooled and don't fool yourself: Products can be listed as "0 grams of trans fats" if they contain 0 grams to less than 0.5 grams of trans fat per serving. You will be able to spot trans fats by reading ingredient lists and looking for the ingredients referred to as "partially hydrogenated oils."

The takeaway is to focus on monounsaturated and saturated fats, and to not skimp on real fats in your daily food choices! Here is an abbreviated list of recommended fats to eat and cook with:

MONOUNSATURATED FATS

- Olives
- Avocados
- Nuts: hazelnuts (or filberts), macadamia nuts, pecans, almonds, pistachios
- Peanuts

SATURATED FATS

- Coconut oil and coconut butter
- Beef brisket and cuts such as rib eye, prime rib or chuck

- Fatty fish such as salmon, mackerel, sardines
- Duck
- Lamb
- Bacon
- Deli meats such as mortadella and salami
- Full fat dairy such as butter and heavy (whipping) cream
- Cooking fats such as ghee, lard, duck fat, lamb fat and chicken fat

If you do not have a dairy sensitivity enjoy FULL FAT dairy such as butter, heavy (whipping) cream and FULL FAT cheeses like feta, Brie and Camembert, blue cheese, Gorgonzola and cheddar. Be aware that some might be higher in carbohydrates than others or higher in protein than others, so I am not saying to eat with abandon, but don't be afraid to eat these wonderful cheeses that you might have been avoiding for years because of the fat. This is not license to put ¼ cup of butter on a fatty steak for no reason other than to eat fat. However, it is license to add fat as you see fit (for flavor, enjoyment and satiety).

The keto advice on fat is to round out your meal with it so you feel you have eaten to satiety. What is satiety? I am sure you have all heard of "Finish your meal and wait 20 minutes before eating more." I know, personally, when I have done this, I have been stuffed 20 minutes later when I took the time to evaluate. Stuffed is not good. I should have stopped even sooner. What are the mechanics of this 20-minute message? One signal comes from your stomach wall stretching to accommodate the meal you are eating. Nerve "stretch receptors" send signals to the brain that the stomach is expanding, and you can begin to taper off and stop eating. Another signal is that a hormone called ghrelin, decreases. Ghrelin is produced when your stomach empties and a hunger message is triggered. Refer often to your mindfulness practice in Step 4 (the hunger scale) until you can put a number to what you are feeling every time you think you are hungry or full. Understanding this scale and the "gut-stretch" response will help you recognize and respect satiety as you go on from here.

THE FINAL STEP IN YOUR TRANSITION TO FULL KETO

ELIMINATE STARCHY AND ROOT VEGETABLES

(LIMIT IF YOU ARE REMAINING LOW CARB)

Okay, the moment of truth. You are ready to transition into becoming fully keto once you accept and practice this final step. This could have been sprung upon you in Step 2 when you cut out grains and legumes, or in Step 3 when you started to limit your carbohydrate intake. But I wanted you to work slowly towards your keto goal so that you would be successful. You are ready now to let go of starchy and root vegetables. Let's define those.

Most starchy vegetables grow below ground. They are loaded with sugar because they feed the greenery that grows above the root. Most people will think of potatoes but also think beets, carrots, parsnips, celeriac, Jerusalem artichokes, shallots, onions and yams. There are others too. Always check the carb counts for a vegetable other than leafy greens until you are comfortable with knowing what you know! Two exceptions to the high-carb, below-ground vegetables are scallions (green onions) and radishes. Above-ground starchy vegetables include winter squashes and corn (which is actually a grain, but many people consider it a vegetable). Pumpkins and tomatoes (which are actually fruits) are higher in carbohydrates but not considered "starchy" and are allowed in very careful quantities. Shiitake mushrooms are an example of an outlier in carbohydrates. They are 10.4 carbohydrates per half cup while most other mushrooms are no more than two carbohydrates per half cup. Ginger and garlic have one carbohydrate for one tablespoon and one clove, respectively, so they certainly can add up in a recipe! My advice is that even if your ultimate goal is not to weigh, measure and track everything you eat, you would be well-advised to look things up at the very beginning. There might be unexpected surprises like those shiitake mushrooms!

The reason "eliminate starchy and root vegetables" is in this final step is because now you are ready to eat to satiety using fat. Up to now, in order to feel full, you may have added a potato to that steak or munched on baby carrots. Now you can concentrate on above-ground vegetables but use ample butter, oil or sour cream with them. Eat a salad using full-fat keto-approved dressings which can be home-made or purchased (read labels carefully). Liberally use olive oil or some other oil that is good for dressing a salad such as nut or avocado oil. If I need something between meals, I find that broth with butter, or a coffee with heavy cream will suffice. Once you increase your fat to satiety, you will very rarely be hungry for a snack.

Regarding broth, you should either be making your own or looking for a packaged one without additives. Read packaged broth (powdered or liquid) ingredients very carefully. You will be surprised at the junk in a lot of them. I use Seitenbacher® Vegetable Broth and Seasoning, which is a powdered bouillon with exceptional no-junk ingredients. Everyone sings the praises of bone broth on keto, and although it has wonderful nutritional and healing properties, you do not HAVE to buy it, make it or eat it.

In considering "fatty coffee," you may have heard of Bullet Proof Coffee® (BPC) in the world of keto. This is actually a registered name of a coffee recipe invented by David Asprey. It has become a term used for any heavy-fat coffee, some using up to ¼ cup of fat per coffee (i.e., two tablespoons coconut oil + two tablespoons butter; two tablespoons heavy cream + one tablespoon butter + one tablespoon MCT oil; etc.). There are so many variations that it is easy to go down a rabbit hole researching them. In the past I used two tablespoons heavy cream + one tablespoon MCT oil, but I ran out of my MCT and now have settled on my two tablespoons of cream per coffee. Once, when I was exploring my dairy-free options I put in pure cocoa butter. A couple of these morning coffees and I am usually good to go until lunch. Personally, I can't get used to the taste of butter in my tea or coffee, but you are welcome to try! If you are going to experiment with anything but straight cream, I suggest you buy a stick frother. A frother will break up the oil slick of fat and create a creamy drink. Do not put your hot beverage into a closed blender and be very careful if you are using an immersion blender.

MCT oil is a topic that sometimes warrants its own scrutinization, but for now, just know that MCT stands for "Medium Chain Triglycerides" and they are not essential to get into ketosis or to remain there. Furthermore, do not purchase any MCT products until you have done full research on your own. If you are set on using MCT oil, then I will tell you that I use David Asprey's Brain Octane. Quite a bit of in-depth research on MCTs (over months) brought me there. I was quite pleased when I found out my own coach also uses that one. Build up slowly. A half of a tablespoon split between two coffees is plenty to start with, otherwise you will surely have, what is affectionately known in the keto world, as "disaster pants." I'll leave that there.

The bottom line of this step is its title: Eat high fat and eliminate (or limit) starchy and root vegetables.

VERY NECESSARY WARNING

High fat in the presence of high carbohydrate intake is dangerous to your heart health. Although you can certainly cut out root and starchy vegetables at any point in your journey, you should not go to the full-fat products as a way of eating if you are not also eating in a very low carb or keto manner. This type of eating – high fat and high carbohydrate – is called obesogenic, causing high blood pressure, fat storage and artery-wall plaque.

MINDFULNESS PRACTICE

Your mindfulness practice here is to repeat the practice in TRANSITIONS STEP 1, but we will take it a little further here. Eat slowly and put your fork down between bites. In order to feel satisfied with the quantity of food you are eating you must SLOW DOWN. Slowing down takes mindful practice and you can easily accomplish this by putting down your fork or food between bites and then actually chewing your food. If you are a fast eater, notice at your next meal whether or not you actually thoroughly chew your food. You will be shocked, I guarantee it. Whenever I am with people who eat more slowly than I do, I always tell myself, "I will not be the first one finished at this table!" Before you even take your first bite take three deep breaths. You can do it quietly so no one else notices. Sit for a moment with your hands in your lap and breathe. Let your senses take in the food. Being mindful and aware of what you are eating will also help you feel more satisfied by the food in front of you. "DIG IN!" does not mean "Shovel it in!" Take your time, eat slowly, chew, swallow and breathe. Survey what is on your plate and take just a few seconds to be grateful for what is in front of you.

When I am not in control of what goes on my plate (like at a restaurant that serves 12 – 16-ounce steaks), I will ask for a container before I even start my meal. I will put half of it in the container from the start. This eliminates picking at the food until it is all gone when I meant only to eat half. At home it is true that taking smaller plates works best on the eye and the brain. You can always take more, but start with what you have, eat slowly and breathe. See if what you initially took is enough. Sometimes after dinner I might have a small number of nuts just to get in the little extra protein, fat and carbohydrates that I might need to top off the day. It makes a nice dessert and puts the final punctuation mark on the meal. You will learn what satiety is – believe me. Things take time. If you are an adult and have been overweight for a long time (look at me – since childhood!) you will have to meet mindfulness and intention at least halfway. I promise, eventually it will become natural for you.

At this point add some slow breathing at various points in your meal – even during the preparation and plating. Just SLOW DOWN. We are always so rushed around food. Just tell yourself that, with each meal, you need the specific vitamins suggested by Mark David which are SD and BE (Slow Down and Breathe). Again, when you sit down with your plate of food in front of you, just take a moment and look at the food and be grateful it is there to nourish you. Take a breath. Eat. Put fork (or food) down. Chew. Swallow. Breathe. You would not think you need to be instructed to do this, until you actually do it and realize that you never do. Centering yourself at this step will prepare you, more than you know, for success with any eating style you plan to follow.

CONGRATULATIONS! YOU ARE NOW FULL KETO!!!

GOOD TO KNOW...

After decades of research, a growing number of experts are questioning the link between high saturated fat intake and heart disease. Current evidence does not clearly support cardiovascular guidelines that encourage low consumption of total saturated fats. Researchers say the relationship between cholesterol and heart disease is a lot more complicated than was once understood. What is now thought to be a more important predictor of risk is the ratio a person has of LDL to HDL, the good cholesterol. There is evidence that, compared with carbohydrates, saturated fat can increase HDL and lower fat deposits in the blood called triglycerides. Triglycerides can be drastically reduced by lowering your carbohydrate intake. Saturated fat also has a relatively neutral effect with regard to raising insulin.

PART THREE
GET THE KRAZINESS OUT OF KETO!

Keto is a fascinating way to eat. It can be very easy, with your calories and food choices coming mainly from protein and fat with non-starchy vegetables on the side, a few nuts and seeds, and, if you are not dairy-free, cream in your coffee and cheese on your burgers. (Yes, it can be that simple!) You can choose to eat from a Yes/No food list which you will find in CHAPTER 10, WAYS OF DOING KETO. It can be no more complicated than that.

OR – It can be difficult either because you make it so, or more likely, you are a lifelong dieter like I am. You are so accustomed to being told what to eat, how much to eat, when to eat and how to eat, that you have lost touch with your own body and don't know when you are hungry or satisfied. You rely on the clock or portion sizes to tell you when to start and stop. You have also lost touch with what makes your body sing and what makes it complain. We are so used to feeling sub par that we may not pick up on cues like eggs not sitting well, peanuts making our hands swell or this vegetable, not that vegetable, causing a low-grade bellyache.

When I first started keto, I wanted to be told what to eat, how much to eat, when to eat and how to eat it. I didn't trust myself. Years of yo-yo dieting taught me that I couldn't. I was so confused because I wanted someone outside of myself to give me the answers. When I was given answers, I questioned them. When I answered my own questions, I doubted the answers. It took a lot of work to learn to make this a lifestyle that I am totally comfortable with now. No charts, no trackers, no books, no nothing except my own wisdom and trust. My hope is that PART 3 of this book does that for you.

Chapter Eight

My Road to Keto

Even though this book talks about everything from emotional issues and habits to my *Granny Keto Transitions Program*™, the light for me switched on when I found keto. I had a very long road to the keto way of eating. In Chapter 1, My Story you saw all the diets I tried, starting with calorie restriction and (sanctioned) diet pills at the age of 13. That road was more like getting lost in a maze of dead ends, traffic circles and street layouts that made no sense. What I am talking about in this chapter is more like the main highway from "here" to "there."

About 10 years ago I was at a doctor's appointment. I was complaining that I was tired all the time. My hair was thinning, and I just couldn't lose weight. The answer was, "Your thyroid tests look fine, but you are fat and that's why you are tired. I'll write a referral to a dermatologist to see about your hair. Oh, and by the way did you notice you have lumps in your neck?" Excuse me, "WHAT? Hell no. What lumps?" My doctor suggested I make an appointment with the endocrinologist in his office, which I did. I had no idea what was going on except that I had a nagging feeling it might have something to do with my thyroid even though my tests always were in a normal range. Who knows if he even did the right tests? I had asked for years about my thyroid as I was "weight-loss resistant" and exhausted to the point where sometimes coming home from work at 5PM, I would have to pull over to the side of the road to sleep before continuing my commute. I would go to the car to sleep during Little League games, high school shows, ceremonies and anything where I might not have been missed while sleeping in the car. My thyroid "numbers" were never a concern to any doctor who saw the results.

The endocrinologist did an antibody test and announced that I had Hashimoto's disease. I had never heard of it and the doctor's reaction was, "We'll just watch you." I did get a biopsy done at that point as well as an ultrasound just to confirm that the nodules were "nothing to worry about" (i.e., not cancer). When I asked the endocrinologist whether I needed medication, his answer was, "We'll just watch you and if the thyroid stops working, we'll deal with it." No explanation about Hashimoto's. I left his office feeling doomed about some awful disease I knew nothing about. That stopped right there. I was not going to allow myself to be an ignorant victim of circumstance. I was too smart and too determined to be that way.

I started combing the Internet for anything I could find. I learned that Hashimoto's disease is an autoimmune condition. Up to that point I never even heard the words "autoimmune condition" and had no idea what it was. I learned that gluten would aggravate autoimmune conditions. I learned that Hashimoto's "sits" at the thyroid so that the thyroid can continue to function – it's almost an overlay and can affect thyroid function, or not – and that it might take years before it affects the functioning of the thyroid. Then from there I Googled "gluten-free" and learned about that. The first thing I read was Dr. William Davis's *Wheat Belly*. Then I Googled "How does a thyroid function, even with Hashimoto's disease?" I found the book *Stop the Thyroid Madness* by Dr. Janie Bowthorpe, as well as the accompanying website by the same name. Then I Googled "Find doctors who encourage gluten-free eating." From there I learned about functional medicine and how functional medicine lab result ranges are entirely different from those of conventional medicine lab-result ranges.

Functional medicine strives to determine the root cause of each disease, particularly chronic diseases such as autoimmune and cardiovascular diseases. Rather than simply making a diagnosis and then determining which drugs or surgery will best treat the condition, functional medicine practitioners dive deep into a patient's history. It is highly personalized and may even include an analysis of one's genetic makeup. Often within a conventional medical practice there may be nurse practitioners who are trained in functional medicine and many times the patient will never even meet the doctor.

I Googled and Googled and Googled until I found functional medicine doctors in my area who were taking patients and my insurance. I made an appointment and when I walked into their offices, I knew I had arrived where I needed to be, especially when I saw they had a stack of *Wheat Belly* books for sale to their patients. It was a practice with functional doctors who specialized in many different areas of medicine. The beauty of functional doctor intake appointments is that the doctor allows up to two hours to meet with the patient. I almost cried as I poured out my heart about how I have been obese and exhausted, and got nothing but blame from my doctors for being lazy, unable to follow diets and that I was, by implication, stupid and lazy. The doctor prescribed a multitude of blood tests including food-sensitivity tests. When I went back for my next appointment, she told me that I did, indeed, have an under-active thyroid (as per functional medicine ranges) and that my weight-loss resistance and exhaustion had a basis in fact, not in innuendos. I never went back to my primary care doctor nor the endocrinologist who stated, "When your thyroid dies, we'll deal with it." Because the practice was so inclusive, I also chose to see an OB/GYN and an orthopedist in the same practice. I never looked back.

My Journey Started with Paleo and an Elimination Diet

The nutritionist on staff started me on an elimination diet based on Paleo. I worked with a functional nutritionist in the practice who guided me into a Paleo way of eating. In addition to being gluten-free, the Paleo lifestyle is all natural and whole foods. This way of eating wasn't a stretch for me and my husband because this is the way we naturally eat. In addition, at this point, both my children were out of the house and on their own, so there was no excuse for buying snack packs of this or that or for using shortcuts to make meals and pack lunches. I fully absorbed the Paleo way of eating, and also learned about, and incorporated, Primal (very similar with a few differences). My husband was totally on board except he continued to have his bread.

I stayed with Paleo for years, but I never lost weight. This included doing a very dedicated Whole 30 program, totally eliminating dairy and artificial sweeteners. For me, that meant no coffee – which I will only take with cream and sweetener – a real commitment, believe me. Again, no weight loss. I would go back for periodic appointments with the functional doctors and nutritionists, and I believe they were secretly rolling their eyes when I insisted that I was not straying – not even one bite – from the Paleo food plan.

I was so distraught that, at one point, I signed up for a wonderful program, Dr. Michelle May's *Mindful Eating*, thinking again, that it was my weakness that was causing the inability to lose weight. I loved the program, and actually do use the mindful practices I learned, but unfortunately it teaches moderation. As I had learned later through keto, my success more often comes from abstention not moderation. Eventually I strayed from everything I had learned from my functional doctors and the Mindful Eating program. At that point I went through another two to three rounds of Weight Watchers. The last time I went to just one meeting and ended it there. I was so hungry I almost chewed my face off on my commute home. I sat and cried and started looking up psychologists who dealt with food addiction. I did see a social worker who was vetted by Tribole and Resch's Intuitive Eating program. Through my work with him I came to believe that it was indeed possible that I couldn't live in the world of moderation. Again, I believed it was all my fault. I believed I was damaged goods.

OPENING MY MIND AND FINDING KETO

During the summer of 2016, a friend of mine was telling me about the Atkins induction phase. I heard "no fruit" and was completely turned off. I'm not going there. Nope. Never. But I did, for the first time, start looking into what low carb means. I read *Weight Loss Zen: An Attitude Adjustment Guide for Keto* by Dixie Vogel. Then I read a book she recommended, *Taking Out the Carbage* by DJ Foodie, then a book that DJ Foodie recommended, *Dr. Gundry's Diet Evolution*. I became a wee bit more open-minded. Then that same friend suggested *Why We Get Fat and What to Do About It* by Gary Taubes, and the rest is history.

Why We Get Fat and What to Do About It changed my life. For the first time I realized it wasn't me. I wasn't being lazy, uncommitted or stupid. **IT WAS THE FOOD. IT WAS THE HORMONES. IT WAS NOT MY FAULT** (to a point, which I will discuss later)! I listened to the book on CD maybe 10 or more times, going over and over the very scientific parts about insulin and hormones, until I could understand every bit of it. One passage meant more to me than any other: "*So long as we believe that people get fat because they overeat, because they take in more calories than they expend, we're putting the ultimate blame on a mental state, a weakness of character, and we're leaving human* *biology out of the equation entirely. . . Do these authors wish to range obesity as a 'behavior problem' among psychiatric instead of metabolic diseases?"* Now, for the first time, I understood that the fruit salads, root vegetables and banana breads made with dates and honey were keeping me fat. The more I tried to be "good" by eating all those real foods instead of candy bars, the deeper I fell into obesity and metabolic disease. Fatty liver, pre-diabetes and sheer exhaustion are not moral diseases, they are metabolic diseases. I am not lazy or stupid. I am metabolically damaged by the foods I thought were good for me. Of course, no diet recommends eating the entire banana bread or fruit bowl, and so I do not blame those diets entirely, whose intentions were good by recommending and supporting whole and good foods. However, with keto and keto principles, it was a start for me, in that the food itself did not fuel endless hunger and cravings, a fact that ultimately helped me to change habits and my mindset.

I learned all I could about keto, hired a coach during the tough times, and found a doctor who was supportive of my keto lifestyle. I do not blame anyone for anything. I have forgiveness because they all – the books, the programs, the doctors – did what they knew to do. Now I know to do what I know to do for myself. I forgive myself too.

SOMETIMES IT IS MORE THAN THE FOOD

I do want to say that because of the years of developing neural pathways with eating certain foods (meaning, "See cookies? Eat." "Bored? Eat." "Upset? Eat." etc.), I still needed to work on habits as much as I needed to work on changing my food choices. This is where I do give credit to the Mindful Eating and Intuitive Eating programs, and also to Geneen Roth's work and others of that ilk. Although moderation was not the right path for me when I started keto, I did learn to face and address many of my poor choices, habits and "head hunger."

Many people do find success with keto just by changing the food that is being eaten. There is no longer the uncontrollable hunger that was due to the high presence of carbohydrates which stimulate the hunger hormones. But, if that person, like me, developed deep and ingrained habits because of that hormone hunger – like eating at night or never being able to have enough food to be satisfied for hours after a meal – it can be hard to change things even without eating the food that triggers hunger hormones. There are also emotional components such as turning to food for years as a substitute for a full and happy life. Or sometimes a habit is just a habit, eating at the movies, while watching TV or joining a partner in a nightly bowl of ice cream.

Yes, there are keto substitutes for all those foods, but again, one of my favorite quotes says: *"Whatever you do, never run back to what broke you."* Personally, I still have problems controlling my eating when keto cookies, breads, cakes and candy are involved. I have friends who do keto and are entirely satisfied with just one piece or one serving of these things, but for them it *is* just the food. Keto helps me tremendously, especially now that I understand how hormones work. I am not hungry all the time, so I am not just rooting around looking for food. However, my emotional baggage is such that sometimes I do have to stop and identify whether I am experiencing "head hunger" and habits or whether I am turning to food to avoid an emotion or activity. I wanted to share this with you so that if you find yourself in a similar situation, you will know that you are not damaged goods. You just need to be a touch more vigilant to stay on the path to well-being.

GOOD TO KNOW....

Very few doctors do a comprehensive thyroid panel. They instead test for TSH (Thyroid Stimulating Hormone) which is produced by the pituitary gland. From this they infer that your thyroid function is high, low or "perfect," and the patient is sent on her way (which is what happened to me!). A comprehensive panel tests the actual thyroid. If you suspect you have low thyroid function (tired all the time, thin hair, fat-loss "resistant"), then be sure to ask for a comprehensive panel that will include the following: Thyroxine (T4), Triiodothyronine (T3), Reverse T3 (rT3), and Thyroid antibodies (both TPO – thyroid peroxidase – and TgAb – Thyroglobulin). Also do your own research and be aware that there are varying acceptable ranges based on whether the ranges are looked at through the eyes of conventional medicine or functional medicine. Just remember that testing TSH and T4 is often not enough!

A SECOND GOOD TO KNOW BECAUSE THIS IS THAT IMPORTANT...

Of course, all of these symptoms below can be caused by a myriad of other things but keep them in mind in case your doctor cannot pinpoint the underlying causes. Double check those thyroid numbers!

COMMON SIGNS OF AN UNDERACTIVE THYROID:

- Tiredness
- Being sensitive to cold
- Weight gain
- Constipation
- Depression
- Slow movements and thoughts
- Muscle aches and weakness
- Muscle cramps
- Dry and scaly skin

- Brittle hair and nails
- Loss of libido (sex drive)
- Pain, numbness and a tingling sensation in the hand and fingers (carpal tunnel syndrome)
- Irregular periods or heavy periods
- Once hypothyroidism has progressed without treatment, signs can also include:
- A low-pitched and hoarse voice
- A puffy-looking face
- Thinned or partly missing eyebrows
- A slow heart rate
- Hearing loss
- Anemia

ADDITIONAL SIGNS OF AN UNDERACTIVE THYROID:

- Elderly people may develop memory problems and depression.

- Children may experience slower growth and development.

- Teenagers may start puberty earlier than normal.

Chapter Nine

Understanding Keto

I want to restate here that keto is not necessary for everyone. With some medical conditions such as glucose-transporter disorder, hypertriglyceridemia and people who suffer from pancreatitis, a person absolutely will not want to follow a keto diet. I am not here, or at any point in this book, suggesting that keto is for everyone. But because many people do consider a keto diet and are able to benefit from this way of eating, my goal is mainly to define it and to help you with ways to successfully follow it.

Here is a short definition: Ketogenic eating ("keto") is a high-fat, adequate-protein, low carbohydrate diet that forces the body to burn fat rather than sugar. It is often referred to as LC/HF, which stands for low carbohydrate/high fat. Eating this way makes the liver convert fat into fatty acids and ketone bodies. An elevated level of ketone bodies in the blood is a state known as ketosis. This is not the same as ketoacidosis. As long as your body produces even a minute bit of insulin, this will not happen to you. Ketoacidosis is a dangerous state in a type 1 diabetic but can be avoided. Especially if you are a type 1 diabetic, you should not proceed with keto unless you are working with a doctor. Keto can be safe if you closely monitor your insulin requirements.

The ketogenic diet was first used to treat difficult-to-control epilepsy in children. The nutritional ketogenic diet most people use is not as severe as the medical ketogenic diet, which has a ratio of 4:1 fat to combined protein and extremely low carbohydrates. When you say, "I'm eating keto," it generally means the nutritional ketogenic diet, which is more likely a 2:1 fat-to-protein ratio. You become a fat burner instead of a sugar burner! (Think of this like a car that either runs or regular gasoline or diesel fuel.) The three macronutrients that you work with are carbohydrates, protein and fat. Micronutrients are the elements of the food, such as vitamins and minerals.

Carbohydrates

The very first thing you do in order to eat keto (and get into ketosis) is to limit your carbohydrates. Carbohydrates is a class of macronutrient. Carbohydrate-rich foods are anything that contain any form of sugar (fruits to candy!) or starch (potatoes, bread and pasta, for instance) which turn into sugar (glucose) in your system. These sugars (whether straight sugar or sugar that has been converted in your body from another food) trigger an insulin response. Insulin is the key that "unlocks" your cell so that the glucose can enter it to provide energy. Excess insulin is responsible for fat storage. Over the years by eating a diet overly rich in high-carbohydrate food, you can develop insulin resistance, meaning that your cells no longer "hear" insulin knocking at the door, and therefore your blood sugar cannot get into your cells to be used for energy. That is why your blood glucose readings will be high when you have type 2 diabetes – it is all that glucose that cannot get into the cells – floating around in your blood. There is also all the extra unused insulin floating around as well.

Very few people eat zero carbohydrates. Some people come very close to that, and this way of eating is called carnivore (animal products and fat only). Some people feel very healthy eating this way. I only mention it here, and it is further discussed in the Appendix. More likely you will be choosing between several levels of carbohydrates and the option to count them as total carbs or net carbs. If you are just getting started and you want to do keto "full on," you might want to start at 20 total carbs and see how you feel. Decide whether it is best for you to go up or down from there or whether you would feel best and do best counting net carbs. The term total carbs means the amount of carbohydrates in a food including fiber and sugar alcohols. The term net carbs means the amount of total carbs in a food item minus the fiber and usually the sugar alcohols as well. Those who believe that neither fiber nor sugar alcohols have any insulin response in the body do not count these carbohydrates in the carbohydrate allowance. They follow the net-carb approach. Because the science on this has not reached definitive conclusions, and actually, because everyone is different in their response to carbohydrate consumption, many who eat keto do not discount the fiber. They count total carbohydrates, but do sometimes factor out all, or half, of the sugar alcohols. One exception to this, seemingly across the board is to count net carbs for an avocado because it is primarily fat and fiber.

If you test your blood glucose levels because you are diabetic or pre-diabetic, you can test before eating and then again two hours after eating certain foods to see if your blood glucose level is the same in both readings. If your level is higher two hours after eating, it means what you have eaten is a food you should stay away from or eat sparingly. This is extremely individual in terms of natural foods, although any processed food such as bread would pretty much tend to raise your levels across the board. Interestingly, if your blood glucose level markedly goes down, it means that you had an insulin response, because the insulin drove down the glucose. It means that the food triggered insulin so you should stay away from the food or eat it sparingly, at least while you are trying to lose weight and heal your body.

COUNTING YOUR CARBS

For people who are less sensitive to carbohydrates (no metabolic disorders or not a lot of weight to lose), you can experiment with allowing yourself a total carbohydrate count of 25 to 30. As time goes on, you can experiment with going higher than that. Your weight loss (or lack of it) and/or blood glucose numbers will tell you if you are on the right path. Another way to "loosen" keto is to not count leafy greens at all. I do that now. I do not count above-ground vegetables and I eat some below-ground vegetables (like carrots) sparingly.

However, please know that counting total carbohydrate grams is the "gold standard" in keto. If you have a lot of healing to do and have, for instance, diabetes, polycystic ovary syndrome (PCOS), inflammation or you have a lot of weight to lose (or on the contrary, you are very close to your weight loss goal) counting total grams of carbohydrates will almost certainly give you the best result.

Please do not get caught up in the net carb myth. A food can have 2 net carbs (sometimes called impact carbs) but be loaded with, for instance, sugar alcohol, fiber and various other starches. For example, the label on PowerBar®'s double chocolate flavor "ProteinPlus Carb Select" bar says it has "2 grams of impact carbohydrates." The Nutrition Facts label on the product says it has 30 grams of total carbohydrates. Unless you are talking about fresh vegetables, net carbs are usually a manufacturer's way of making you think they are inconsequential when, in fact, many of the subtracted carbohydrates do impact blood sugar and insulin. If you decide to go the net-carb route, be very aware of stalls in weight loss, how your body feels and whether your blood glucose is affected if you test regularly.

My own carb-counting system combines net and total carbohydrates and I have had many clients who are successful with that. I call it Granny Keto's "Hybrid System" for counting carbs. In a nutshell, I count total carbs in any food that is not an above-ground vegetable or is an avocado (which is mostly fat and fiber). For vegetables I count the net carbs and add it to the total, for a combined total of 20 carbs.

PROTEIN

I am going to repeat here, almost verbatim, the section on protein in *GRANNY KETO TRANSITIONS PROGRAM™* STEP 4 (CHAPTER 6) because some readers may have skipped ahead to these chapters on keto without carefully reading that one. I do not want you to miss any part of the protein lesson in that step. If you have already carefully read CHAPTER 6, so much the better. A double dose of learning about protein will double your chances of success!

MODERATE – BUT DO NOT FEAR – YOUR PROTEIN INTAKE. When you are fully keto, please understand that you are not going to be eating unlimited amounts of protein. But you should not be worried about eating too much. Even when eating the carnivore diet (please see Appendix) which is animal products only, you will still be listening to your hunger signals. Protein triggers feedback on satiety more efficiently than carbohydrates. Pay attention and you will not be having "all-you-can-eat" quantities of meat. At the time of publication of this book, no organization has established a firm upper limit on what might constitute "too much" protein in a person's diet. Also, in a healthy individual, the body will safely rid itself of unneeded protein.

Protein is an essential nutrient. Proteins are the building blocks of cells and muscles, and they are essential for brain function and other functions, such as healing cuts and wounds. The body will recycle much of its protein and you do not need to consume large quantities to have a healthy body. In fact, by a process called gluconeogenesis, in which the liver can convert amino acids (from protein) into glucose, the liver may produce a little too much glucose, which could impact insulin. This, however, is usually not a supply-driven process. It is mostly a demand-driven process, meaning that it doesn't automatically happen if you eat a lot of protein. It happens if and when your body needs glucose. The issue of the liver converting protein into excessive glucose as a supply-driven process tends to happen more in people with very severe insulin resistance or difficult-to-control diabetes.

Another thing to consider if you tend to eat a lot of protein is that protein contains a lot of phosphorus which is a stimulant. As a result, you will find you might not sleep well after a heavy protein dinner!

Grams of protein means the number of grams of protein that is in a food, not the weight of the food in grams. For example, three ounces of ground chuck, cooked, weighs 85 grams and contains 22 grams of protein. The same three ounces (85g) of cooked bacon, contains 9 grams of protein. This is a question that comes up frequently when people are new to keto. Not to worry – just make sure you are measuring the correct thing! There are various calculations and formulas based on height, body mass, or other factors such as BMR (Basal Metabolic Rate) and TDEE (Total Daily Energy Expenditure). However, human beings are not machines, and calculators should not rule your lifestyle.

When you are beginning keto or low carb eating, the only metric you have to pay attention to is your carbohydrate count. However, if you want to follow keto you will see a lot of references to your macros. Macro is an abbreviation for macronutrient, referring to carbohydrates, proteins or fats. When you hear the term macro in a keto discussion, that refers to the grams you are allowed for each category. Although I do want you to be informed about what you are reading, I do not agree with the extremely low protein allotment that most keto sites suggest. As of the publishing of this book there is a new face of keto that is popping up among researchers and social media influencers. The new wisdom is to do just what I am telling you here: Do not severely moderate protein, and the older you are, the more you need to add to your diet.

One simple (and older, but prevalent) calculation for keto-protein allotment is 45.5 grams per 5' of height, then every inch over 5' multiply by 2.3 and add it to 45.5. There are other formulas that may include body mass, BMR, and TDEE. If you are young, an athlete and not metabolically challenged in any way, you can have more than whatever that calculation is. If you are not losing weight, not getting into ketosis or have conditions such as non-alcoholic fatty liver disease, are severely insulin resistant, have type 2 diabetes, etc., you may want to work within that calculated number and pay close attention to the "incidental" protein that I talk about below.

The protein allotment that I prefer and have suggested to my clients since being in practice, is one that is more realistic (and backed by research), which is 1.2 to 1.7 grams per kilogram of "reference" body weight. The reference weight is not your goal weight necessarily, but what is an average weight for your height. For instance, I am 5'4" and my "reference" body weight is approximately 140 pounds (64 kg). I got this by using a standard BMI chart, looking up my height and then picking the number that falls at the high end of a "normal" BMI, which is 24. (We can split hairs here: normal is up to 24.9 but then the math gets too hard!) My protein allowance should fall between 76.8 to 108.8 grams of consumed protein (not grams of weight).

What does this look like for meals? When you start out, you will probably be eating three meals a day. I recommend STRONGLY that you limit yourself to three adequate meals that cut out any need for snacking. Start with that and arrange your protein grams accordingly. The best way to approach this is to split your protein fairly evenly between these three meals. Divide your day into three meals, which comes out to about 30 grams of protein per meal. This is main-course protein. You will also be eating "incidental" protein in vegetables, coffee cream, cheese, nuts and seeds. When I started keto, I paid no attention to limiting protein. As I stopped losing weight, it was the first thing that my coach and I looked at. I cut slightly back on protein, mostly paying more attention to the "incidentals" rather than cutting too far back on my main meal proteins. I am not telling you this to discourage you, but to acknowledge that learning your sweet spot with protein can be difficult, but you can do it! The biggest "struggle" was just mindfulness – paying attention to what I was eating and learning protein counts of food. When I did count macros, just to get things in line, I did look things up and I was so surprised to find that fish and shellfish and other lean protein pack a lot of protein into each serving size. As long as you are eating good quality protein, don't worry too much about that. It is unlikely that a woman is going to overeat protein (in fact, most women are not getting enough!) and you don't have to run back and forth to your food scale to shave off an ounce of something. You need to make this a lifestyle and not a diet!

Eat good quality protein and pay attention to your hunger signals. If you are still afraid of protein after all you have read on social media, and want to avoid overeating, engage in *sequential eating* as coined by Dr. Robert Cywes. Again, some people call this putting in a speed bump. Take what you feel is an adequate portion of food and divide it onto two plates. Put the plate in front of you that you are going to eat and put the other plate either in the middle of the table or on a kitchen counter. Finish what is in front of you, then see if you want the rest. This is a great mindfulness practice to use. Do not take 3 ounces of protein (the standard "deck-of-cards" or "palm-of-your-hand" sized portion) and divide that. Take something substantially more to start. If you are still hungry and want to eat more, EAT MORE!!! Choose protein sources where the fat is part of the protein such as chicken thighs with the skin, egg yolks (not just the whites) and steak that is marbled or has the fat layer around it, like a good rib eye. These choices will automatically align protein and fat recommendations and will keep you full longer on less food!

Don't make yourself crazy with macros but rather, really begin to listen to your body. Furthermore, pick protein options that come packaged with their own fat (marbled and higher fat meats, chicken legs with the skin on, full fat dairy, oily fish like salmon and sardines, etc.). When you get to Dancing with Low Carb and Keto (Chapter 13) you will find your sweet spot with protein. Just a little more than some might recommend for keto might make you feel better, energy-wise and digestion-wise. This might make the difference between being successful or not.

Remember these two concepts when choosing how much protein to eat: We are not machines and must eat according to what makes us feel best. For some, it might be a little more protein and a little less fat than a standard macro calculation would have you eating. DO NOT FEAR protein. Gluconeogenesis is almost always a demand-driven process and not a supply-driven process.

Fat

The last macronutrient is Fat. The rule here is to eat to satiety. There are various ratios. For instance, when the ketogenic diet is used to treat and control epilepsy, a 4:1 ratio of fat to protein is prescribed. This means that for every gram of protein you eat (not the weight but the amount of protein in the food), you eat four times as many grams of fat. You will not be eating this ratio. A comfortable ratio for "regular" eating is a minimum of 1:1, but most people settle in at 2:1. Even at the 1:1 ratio, some people starting keto find it difficult to eat so much fat, especially those who grew up in the fat-free era, or even younger people who have been fed the myth of fat-free, most often from mothers who were always on a diet.

You may also worry about so much fat if you do not have a gallbladder or have one but are having gallbladder issues. There are two ways to approach this, but ultimately the extra fat will not burden your system. The first is to take digestive enzymes that will help your gallbladder (or system, if you no longer have a gallbladder) process fats. I do not have a gallbladder and took these enzymes my first couple of months. I never had a problem. The other thing to do is to slowly increase your fats, instead of diving right in.

FAT – AND ESPECIALLY SATURATED FAT – DOES NOT CAUSE HEART DISEASE. The sugar and carbohydrates in your diet cause hardening of the arteries. HONEST.

As suggested above, the easiest way to start to increase your fat intake is to go for fattier cuts of meat. Eat less turkey deli meat because it is highly insulinogenic, which means it raises your insulin which makes you fat; it is also too lean. Instead, choose deli meats like roast beef, corned beef, salami and pastrami. Eat less boneless, skinless chicken breasts, and instead prepare more meals using chicken thighs with skin. Instead of lean ground beef, purchase ground beef with a higher fat profile (such as 80% meat and 20% fat). It will be cheaper too, and don't drain the fat! Enjoy ribeye steak and a nice, marbled chuck roast instead of lean sirloin and London broil. Eat more fatty fish like salmon and mackerel. Don't feel you have to eat cod or other white fish because they are leaner.

Move to full-fat dairy. Yes, I said FULL FAT. That means sour cream to top your steak, butter to top your vegetables, heavy cream in your coffee, REAL cheese and bacon. No need to weigh, measure or count out the pieces. If you enjoy it, just eat it. And NO – you do not have to eat bacon or any pork products on keto. But you can if you want. Avocados, other fats and some oils are perfect ways to add to your fat intake. So, in a nutshell, if you are following conventional macro recommendations, 5% of your caloric intake will be from carbohydrates, 20% to 25% will be from protein and 75% to 80% will come from fat.

KETOSIS AND MEASURING KETONES

Ketosis, not to be confused with ketoacidosis, will be your metabolic state where your body's energy supply comes from ketone bodies in the blood, which are produced when you metabolize fat, converting fatty acids into ketones. When you are in ketosis, you will have measurable ketones (generated by fatty acids in the liver) and you will become a fat burner, with these ketones providing energy to your brain and the rest of your body.

There are three types of ketones: acetone, acetoacetate (AcAc) and Beta-Hydroxybutyrate (BHB). Each is measured differently, in the breath, urine and blood, respectively. The breath (using a "breathalyzer") measures the ketones you have used, the urine measures the ketones you are producing, and the blood is the gold standard, measuring how many ketones you have available to use.

There is a bit of controversy on the urine strips. This is because when you first start, it is great feedback to see that you are producing ketones. The problem lies in the fact that as you are in ketosis for longer periods of time and your body gets used to producing and using ketones, there aren't as many left over to "spill" into your urine. Many people go berserk, when all of a sudden, their sticks go back to beige and they no longer pee pink or purple. They think they are doing something wrong and start to cut their macronutrients back to practically nothing – or – they give up just when things are actually at their best. Another flaw with these sticks is that you might "pee purple" (the highest level) but it might be that you are dehydrated. When you drink water to correct this, the next day your color might drop back down to a light pink. Then you worry you are losing your ketosis edge (not true!).

For the $10 or so that a bottle of "pee-sticks" cost, it is a great way to find encouragement at the beginning of your journey. That being said, there are very successful people who have never measured their ketone levels by any manner.

Being Fat Adapted

You might hear the term fat adapted. This means that your body has shifted over to fat burning and that you are in ketosis most of the time. You can eat some foods (or quantities of food) that might knock you out of ketosis (under .5 on the blood meter). However, if you have been in ketosis for a while, your body always prefers fat for its fuel. Very little glucose will be available for your body to burn and so your body will continue to burn and produce ketones even though they may register very low. After a day or two of eating keto, you will get back to a good level of ketosis again. The better fat adapted you are, the less time it will take to start producing ketones again.

The Keto Flu and Electrolytes

The next thing that you will have to work with, besides balancing your macronutrients, is electrolyte balance. Some people will experience the "Keto Flu" the first week or so of starting keto. The symptoms might be:

- Fatigue
- Headache
- Irritability
- Difficulty focusing ("brain fog")
- Lack of motivation
- Dizziness
- Sugar cravings
- Nausea

You can usually spare yourself this experience if you have adequate amounts of three electrolytes: sodium, magnesium and potassium. Also, people who have gradually built up to keto using my Transitions steps are less likely to experience the keto flu, which is just a shock to your system from the sudden decrease in carbohydrate intake.

I look at a carbohydrate as a sponge. On the Standard American Diet (SAD) you can consume upwards of 300 grams of carbohydrates or more per day. When you start keto, you will be starting with 20 grams of carbohydrates. Imagine those 300 sponges wringing out all the water they hold. You will be releasing a lot of fluid when you start keto, and you will not be eating any more sponges. Thus, at the beginning of eating keto you might feel you are losing only water weight. Eventually your kidneys will find their sweet spot for perfect functioning. At that point you will know for certain you are losing fat and not just water. And know this: salt follows the water. When you are eating keto, you must replenish your salt (and water!). It is recommended that you have 4g to 5g a day of salt. This is two teaspoons straight salt if you are not salting your food. This recommendation is *only* if you are following keto. Do not salt that hamburger if you are putting it in a bun with ketchup and relish. The same applies for the fat recommendations. Keep in mind that these numbers and recommendations should only be followed if your total carbs or net carbs are in the vicinity of 20!

Even when you are past the "keto flu" stage at the beginning, you may still experience leg cramps or some other symptoms such as fatigue and dizziness. This is because you still need to keep up your electrolytes even when you are well into ketosis and are fat-adapted. When you go to keto sites you may read a lot about leg cramps at night and people who jump out of bed and drink pickle juice or guzzle salt straight out of the shaker. I have done both myself when I haven't been careful during the day! (A word about salt: purchase pink, sea or gray salt. Table salt sometimes is mixed with anti-caking and bleaching agents.)

Magnesium and potassium can also be flushed from your system with your super-duper functioning kidneys. There are many people who do not take supplements because they are careful to get what they need from the foods they eat. One magnesium-rich food which is allowed on keto is dark chocolate, if it is low in sugar. Avocado, nuts and seeds, fatty fish and leafy greens are other sources of magnesium. However, most people are deficient in magnesium even if they eat these foods and so a supplement is usually recommended. There are different types of magnesium, each offering a different benefit to the body. My doctor recommended chelated magnesium glycinate which is what I take as my magnesium supplement. Do your own research or talk with your doctor.

You should be consuming up to 4000 mg of potassium a day but try not to get it through supplements. An overage of potassium can be dangerous so try to get what you need from foods – the same list as the magnesium. If you have an avocado and a nice helping of Swiss chard or spinach with one of your meals, you will easily approach what you need. Add tomatoes and Brussels sprouts, and you are good to go. (And by the way, sugar cravings can be caused by the need for potassium so make sure you keep up with that mineral!)

SUMMARY

There is so much to learn about keto, but remember the following:

- Keep carbs low
- Eat adequate protein
- Eat high fat to satiety
- Address your electrolytes: sodium, magnesium and potassium

Good to Know...

Twenty years ago, a little boy named Charlie Abrahams developed difficult-to-control epilepsy. As a last resort, his parents turned to the medically supervised ketogenic diet. The diet worked and Charlie became seizure-free. He remained on the diet for 5 years and then returned to a normal diet. He's now in his twenties and has remained seizure- and medication-free. The Charlie Foundation for Ketogenic Therapies was founded in 1994 to provide information about diet therapies for people with epilepsy, other neurological disorders and tumorous cancers. New applications of the ketogenic diet for cancer, autism, ALS, Parkinson's, early-onset Alzheimer's disease, diabetes and traumatic brain injury have emerged. Variations of the ketogenic diet for these disorders are being developed. For more information visit www.charliefoundation.org.

CHAPTER TEN

WAYS OF DOING KETO

There are many ways to do keto. This is the most challenging part of being on a keto diet. It is not the food restrictions at all, but that there is no prescribed way of eating. Nothing is being spoon fed to you. This is a double-edged sword in that if you have a long dieting history like me, you are accustomed to being told "eat this, not that," "count this, not that," "think this, not that." Keto is truly a way of eating where you must listen to your body. This is true even if you choose to count macros (your allotted portion of fat, protein and carbohydrate) and choose to stop eating for the day when your digital counter tells you so. Your ability to figure out your hunger signals might be stunted but you still must listen to your body to figure out which foods and quantities make you feel best.

We are so out of touch with our bodies because of mealtimes dictated by the clock, our social lives and ceaseless bad habits. We no longer know our hunger and fullness signals, a skill which is essential for doing any method of keto. As noted above, some people will still count macros and will only eat according to the digital calculations. However, it is more prudent to learn how you feel about the quantity or type of food you are eating in order to make the keto experience more natural and lifelong. CHAPTER 12, THE HUNGER SCALE (and the Mindfulness Practice in CHAPTER 6), will help you to home in on your hunger and satiety signals.

What follows is an explanation of "basic keto" as well as two of the popular ways of doing keto. These are eating from a "Yes/No" list and counting Macros (protein, fat and carbohydrates). There are several other ways to do keto and you might even develop your own. You can find these in the APPENDIX. These additional ways of doing keto are probably not an exhaustive list, but they are a good representation of the choices a person doing keto will have. My hope is that this will clear up some of the confusion as you hear the various terms on social media, from Facebook to arguments on Reddit!

BASIC KETO

When you first start to learn about keto (as I did by reading *Why We Get Fat and What to Do About It* by Gary Taubes, *Keto Clarity* by Jimmy Moore and Eric Westman, and about a half dozen informative keto cookbooks), you will learn about the basics of keto, which are: "Keep carbs low, moderate protein, and don't fear good fats." Most basic keto instructions will tell you to keep your carbohydrates to 20 grams, total or net. From there you will be instructed to keep your protein grams to about 50 for women and 80 for men (WAY TOO LOW!! See discussions in CHAPTERS 6 and 9). Then you are encouraged to eat at least double that in fat (100 grams of fat for a woman and 160 grams of fat for a man). Because we are not machines or computers, it is impossible to measure these needs to a fault, as digital calculations would have you believe is possible. At the most liberal, you would be instructed to keep your carbs to 20, total or net, and eat protein and fat to satiety. This is where newcomers often get into trouble. If you don't eat in response to hunger, how on earth are you ever going to know what it means to "eat when you are hungry and stop when you are satisfied?" For instance:

- Eating lunch during an assigned lunch hour;
- Eating at night because it has always been a habit;
- Not stopping when you start to feel you have had enough;
- You don't have a sense of being full;
- You eat until the food is gone; or
- You eat mindlessly.

Keep in mind that if you are coming from a Standard American Diet (SAD) or a cultural diet where you consume a lot of grains and legumes, you will probably lose weight and improve your health just by cutting down the carbohydrates and sugars. However, long term, you will also want to pay attention to the following:

- Keep your carbohydrate count to the vicinity of 20 carbs (total or net).
- Moderate your protein intake (this is not an all-you-can-eat-until-you-burst steak diet).
- Keep your healthy fats high (and healthy for keto includes saturated fats).

CHOOSING FROM YES/NO FOOD LISTS

The easiest way to do "basic" keto is to keep to 20 grams of carbohydrates, total or net, and eat from a Yes/No list. There are several of these all across the web. Some say no nuts, seeds or nut flours, but a dairy choice like yogurt is okay; others will say yes to nuts and seeds but might outlaw any form of dairy (because of its inflammatory properties). Some will put limits on certain foods even within a Yes/No list.

Wherever you get these lists from, be aware of their origins. For instance, Dr. Eric Westman's "Page Four" list (based on recommendations from Dr. Atkins and Jackie Eberstein, RN) is very popular in some keto cultures. He limits foods and excludes some because of the health conditions and eating habits of these patients who may be in dire circumstances. It is not meant to be the bible on what to eat or not to eat on a ketogenic diet. However, hundreds, if not thousands, of people have been successful with weight loss and reversing medical conditions, and do not find the list restrictive. Whatever the list, just changing your eating habits and going low on carbohydrates will probably be enough to get the weight loss going.

Here is my suggested Yes/No List as a guide to what foods are keto and what foods are not keto. The short list is really the answer to: What can I eat on keto? What do I get at the grocery store?

THE SHORT LIST

YES LIST

- Any animal protein (the fattier the better!)
- Full-fat dairy
- Healthy fats
- Green leafy vegetables and above-ground vegetables
- Nuts and seeds
- Berries

NO LIST

- Sugars or processed foods containing sugars
- Grains or processed foods containing grains
- Legumes or processed foods containing legumes
- Starchy vegetables or processed foods containing starchy vegetables
- Fruit (except berries) or fruit juice (except small quantities of lemon and lime juices)

THE LONG LIST

(Disclaimer: This longer list is an amalgamation of many keto lists you can find in any book or any website. It is not a direct copy of any one list. If it resembles any author's list directly, that is because it is a standard and common keto foods list.)

ANIMAL PROTEIN

- Beef (all cuts)
- Beef deli meats (but check for the carb counts — some may be high if there are added sugars or fillers)
- Pork (all cuts)
- Pork deli meats (but check carb counts — some may be high if there are added sugars or fillers)
- Beef and Pork "snack" items such as:
  - Pork rinds/skins
  - Pepperoni slices
  - Bacon (sugar used in the curing process will burn off but do not have sugared bacon such as maple-flavored; just buy plain)

- Eggs (any kind)
- Lamb
- Veal
- Other meats such as venison
- Chicken (preferably dark meat with skin)
- Turkey (preferably dark meat with skin)
- Duck
- All Fish
- All Shellfish

SALAD GREENS

- Arugula
- Bok Choy
- Cabbage (all varieties)
- Chard
- Endive
- Greens (all varieties such as beet, collard, mustard and turnip)
- Kale
- Lettuce (all varieties)
- Radicchio
- Radishes (although this is technically a root vegetable, it is often included in the leafy green category)
- Scallions (spring/green onion) (same comment as radishes, above)
- Spinach
- Sprouts
- Watercress

FRESH HERBS

- Basil
- Chives
- Parsley
- Cilantro
- Thyme
- ALL other fresh herbs
- Dried herbs can be used but if you are using in excess of one tablespoon in a recipe, be aware that the carbohydrates add up.

FIBROUS AND CRUCIFEROUS VEGETABLES

- Artichokes
- Asparagus
- Bell peppers (all colors)
- Broccoli
- Brussels sprouts
- Cauliflower
- Celeriac (use sparingly – this is a root vegetable)
- Celery
- Chayote
- Green beans (string beans)
- Jicama (use sparingly — this is a root vegetable)
- Mushrooms (warning: Shiitake mushrooms are very high carb!)
- Okra
- Onions (use sparingly — this is a root vegetable)
- Pumpkin
- Snow peas
- Sugar snap peas
- Summer squash
- Tomatoes (high carb, be careful to limit — these are actually fruit!)
- Turnip (use sparingly — this is a root vegetable)
- Zucchini

You might ask here why some root vegetables are included while others are not. Some of these are used for seasoning (such as garlic and ginger) and are not the main attraction. Others, such as Jicama and turnip are on this list as they are not as high in sugar as other root vegetables, but you still have to pay attention to the carb count and eat them sparingly or not often.

FATTY FRUIT

- Avocado
- Olives

CHEESE

- Use full-fat ONLY and preferably raw cow, goat, sheep cheeses
- This includes hard cheeses (i.e., sliceable like cheddar, gouda)
- Semi-soft (i.e., Brie, blue, Gruyere)
- Soft (i.e., ricotta, cottage, farmers, cream)
- Stay away from processed cheese such as American

CREAM

- Use full fat ONLY
- Heavy (whipping) cream
- Light, or table, cream
- Sour cream
- No half & half; no condensed or evaporated milk

HEALTHY FATS AND OILS

- Butter
- Coconut oil and coconut butter
- Lard, tallow, chicken fat, duck fat, bacon fat
- Avocado oil
- Olive oil and nut oils for cold use (they are unstable when heated)
- Bottled dressings are acceptable if the carb count is 1 gram per serving:
  - Blue cheese
  - Ranch
  - Caesar

MAYONNAISE

- Homemade is best. If you buy avocado or olive oil mayo, make sure the ingredients are not really canola or soybean oil dressed up as avocado or olive oils.

BERRIES

- There are many kinds of berries and they are all allowed on keto. However, keep your portions small and eat them not more often than once a day. You can even use the tarter berries such as cranberries, but if you must sweeten them you will want to pick from the list of sugar alternatives or artificial sweeteners.

NUTS AND SEEDS AND THEIR BUTTERS

- If you are going to eat nuts and seeds, be VERY careful with your measurements and realize that there are also carbohydrates and proteins in these foods in addition to the fat. If you can't control yourself, then don't start with them. Even if you can control yourself, be careful. Be sure to have only unsweetened nut butters and look for those with only 1 or 2 ingredients (i.e., the nut or seed and salt).

PICKLES

- Dill
- Half-sour
- Sour
- NO bread & butter or other pickles with sugar

CONDIMENTS

- Lemon and lime juice (Watch the carb count. One tablespoon = 1 carb.)
- Yellow mustard (or any mustard with no sugar)
- Coconut aminos (This product is similar to soy sauce but watch the carbs.)
- Salt and pepper
- Vinegar
- Dill relish
- Sugar-free sweet relish
- Low carb or sugar-free versions of ketchup and barbeque sauce. There are many keto recipes for these, or you can use the bottled brands based on your own preferences for consuming artificial sweeteners.

Just because foods are on this list does not mean that you can eat them with abandon. At the very least, you must keep track of your carbohydrate totals. I have my own carbohydrate system (the Granny Keto hybrid system of counting carbs), which is net carbs for avocados and green leafy and other above-ground vegetables added to the total carbs for all other foods. I total these to equal a grand total of 20 carbohydrates. If you are exceptionally sensitive to carbohydrates, you may want to count only total carbohydrates no matter what the source.

COUNTING MACROS

Many people refer to this as the "gold standard" of doing a ketogenic diet. I don't disagree, but yet I strongly do. Knowledge is power. I believe that in order to be successful you have to define what each of these macronutrients is: carbohydrate, protein and fat, and know what you are aiming for (either in finite quantities such as 20 grams of carbohydrates, 80 to 100 grams of protein, and anywhere from 100 to 200 grams of fat) or in percentages based on calorie intake for your body weight (for example, 5% carbohydrates, 15% to 20% protein and 75% to 80% fat). However, to take these values as absolute, as many do, has three glaring errors:

We are not machines. Even if you get out your calculators and figure BMR (Basal Metabolic Rate: The estimation of the number of calories you would burn even if you never got out of bed in the morning); TDEE (Total Daily Energy Expenditure: The estimation of the number of calories you burn based on your exercise and activities); and any other rates (using body fat percentage, quality of sleep, etc.), notice the word ESTIMATION. Every person is different and calculating these, and ultimately your macros, is a fuzzy estimation at best, not an exact science.

When you eat to your macros you run the risk of never truly learning what feels best in your body or recognizing your hunger and satiety signals. It is a very external locus-of-control method (see CHAPTER 13, DANCING WITH LOW CARB AND KETO, for more on locus of control). You rely on outside sources to tell you when to stop eating or what foods to eat at any given meal. I am all for planning out your day, but what happens when you have planned one food to fit your daily macros, but it is not available, or you just don't want it? This is not the case for everyone, and I am not saying it is, but it reminds me too much of prescribed diet plans. If some of these diet companies folded tomorrow, there would be hundreds of thousands of dieters who would immediately gain weight because they never really learned about their bodies and their needs.

There is no allowance for differences in calories or macros between different qualities of food. Whether or not you are in the organic or grass-fed, pasture-raised camp, there is mounting evidence that these foods are more nutrient dense than conventionally grown fruits and vegetables or feedlot-raised animals, which may affect calorie and macro counts. Further, we do not know whether GMOs ultimately affect the calories of certain foods. My two cups of organic, non-GMO lettuce might not have the same calories (or macros) as a cup of conventional lettuce. My four ounces of grass-fed beef might not have the same calories (or macros) as feedlot beef. I am not standing on one soap box or the other here, I am just pointing out that there is no exact science in figuring macros when we also consider the quality of the foods we eat.

Good to Know...

Macro(nutrient) is a keto buzzword, but it is also important to know about Micronutrients. The term micronutrient refers to vitamins and minerals which can be divided into macro minerals, trace minerals and water- and fat-soluble vitamins. Vitamins are needed for energy production, immune function, blood clotting and other functions. Minerals benefit growth, bone health, fluid balance and other processes. It is best to get these from food rather than supplements. There can be toxicity problems if you are getting too much of any of these. Water-soluble vitamins are B1, B2, B3, B5, B6, B7, B9, B12 and Vitamin C. Fat-soluble vitamins are A, D, E and K. Macro minerals are Calcium, Phosphorus, Magnesium, Sodium, Chloride, Potassium, and Sulfur. Trace minerals are Iron, Manganese, Copper, Zinc, Iodine, Chromium, Cobalt, Fluoride and Selenium.

Chapter Eleven

Questions and Myths

Here are questions that I have been asked both by my clients and through the "Ask Granny" feature on my earlier website.

- *Do I have to eat anything made with coconut, bacon, heavy cream, coffee, tea or anything else that is popular in social media posts?* There are no required foods on keto. PERIOD. This includes coffee, tea and all renditions of coffee and tea. The reason that this question pops up so often is that there are certain foods that are popular on keto, but they are not requirements.

- *Do I have to fast?* Absolutely not. Because of some health benefits that have been found with fasting (a correction in blood glucose, improvement with fasting insulin and autophagy, to name a few) and due to the comprehensive research done by Dr. Jason Fung who has made access to all this information available at the layperson's fingertips, the information on fasting has become mainstream information especially for the keto community. That is why there is so much talk about it. You do not have to fast to be on a ketogenic diet. Furthermore, once you are on a successful keto diet your hunger and fullness hormones (ghrelin and leptin, respectively) will be corrected. They will be brought into normal range because of the decrease in insulin production which had been kept elevated due to a high carbohydrate intake. With these hormones no longer wreaking havoc in your body, you are satisfied with less food and with eating less often. It is not unusual to want to eat only one or two meals a day. Instead of three meals and two snacks (or 6 small meals) a day you might automatically fall into an intermittent fasting pattern. But no, you do not need to force fasting on yourself.

- *Do I have to eat organic? Do I have to eat grass-fed and pasture-raised meats?* No, you do not. Although keto definitely is based on whole healthy foods you do not have to eat organic and grass-fed, pasture-raised foods. There is no controversy over some of the benefits of these foods. Eliminating foods produced with harmful pesticides is one such benefit. Also, many organic fruits and vegetables are considered more nutrient dense than conventionally grown produce. This is because organic crops are rotated and soils naturally amended to grow strong and healthy plants, quashing a "gang's all here" environment for pests. With regard to produce, nutrient density refers to amounts of vitamins, minerals and phytonutrients. Phytonutrients are the thousands of chemicals, some of which are not even known yet, that are produced by strong healthy plants and which are valuable to one's health. Totally steering clear of political and ethical arguments with regard to grass-fed and pasture-raised animals, as opposed to feedlot-sourced animals, it has been shown that animals from these sources help support healthy blood sugar levels, contain electrolytes and help fight cancer because the meat contains roughly twice the amount of conjugated linoleic acid (CLA) compared to grain-fed beef. CLA is considered to be one of the strongest nutrients that can defend against cancer. Grass-fed meat contains more healthy fats (up to six times more omega-3 fatty acids than grain-fed beef), contains less bacteria and can decrease your risk of heart disease because of high antioxidants such as vitamin E, high amounts of omega-3 fatty acids and a high CLA profile. (Please see Dr. Anthony Gustin at PerfectKeto.com, for further easy-to-understand material on this, including what the label "organic" really means.) However, although you do not need to eat organic and grass-fed foods, if your budget permits, you may want to include more of these foods in your diet.

- An ancillary question: *Won't eating keto be expensive, even if I don't eat organic and grass-fed? What do you mean, money left over in my budget?* When you first eat keto, you may have a few weeks of high grocery bills, but this is only temporary. First of all, when you start any new way of eating your grocery bills go up because you are probably not eating foods that as a rule you keep in your house. That could be anything from packaged foods and shakes for something like Slimfast®, to what seems like tons of fresh produce for something like Paleo. The difference with keto is that your appetite will naturally decrease, and you will be buying less food. I always like to give this example: Before keto, my husband would buy two 1-pound (at least) ribeye steaks to go on the grill for our dinner (just the two of us). After a few months on keto, he would buy one 1-pound steak for the two of us. Now he buys the one steak, he eats half, and I eat about 2/3^{rds} of my half and use the rest on top of some salad for lunch the next day. Now we find that we have that "left-over" money in our budget. As a result, more and more often we have the money to buy the organic, grass-fed, pasture-raised and wild-caught versions of the food we eat. And don't forget, you will not be spending money on all that fast-food, take-out and snack food you used to eat!

- *Do I have to weigh and measure my food? Do I have to count macros?* NO and NO. Let me tell you a story that cemented this way of eating for me: When I was on Weight Watchers, we could have baked potatoes, but the Points were based on a 10-ounce raw potato. I laid my kitchen scale inside my purse but across the top so that when I put the potato down, I could prove I wasn't shoplifting. I took loose russet potatoes one by one and weighed them to find the 10-ounce ones. I eventually got proficient at just picking up a potato, and right on the money, know it would be 10 ounces. I did this at restaurants to weigh meat and fish portions (and oh my, the applause I got in the Weight Watchers meeting room for doing that!). Granted, that was a little obsessive, but welcome to my world, as I am sure many of yours. Study Dancing with Low Carb and Keto (CHAPTER 13) and see how you can start to learn to let go of the weighing, measuring and tracking. It will make a world of difference in your life, I promise.

- *Do I have to count calories?* On one level the answer is the same NO as "Do I have to count macros?" The type of calorie matters more than the number of calories (in the short run). By this I mean that 100 calories of broccoli or butter do not deliver the same nutrition to your body as 100 calories of potato chips or chocolate cake. With the broccoli and butter, you will have little to no insulin response. With the potato chips and chocolate cake, you will have a rise in insulin, your fat storage hormone. As long as you begin to decrease your carbohydrates and increase your fats, eat only when hungry and stop when satisfied, you will have successful weight loss and maintenance. That is why many keto proponents totally dismiss the "CICO" theory of "Calories In – Calories Out." In the long run, however, YES, calories ultimately matter. Eating 1,000 extra calories of fat, for instance, may be more than your body needs or can burn, and you will not burn your body fat. Chances are, however, if you are eating that many extra calories (even the "good" ones) then you are not listening to your hunger and satiety signals. Get good at that, and you will never have to be concerned.

- *Do I have to eat fat bombs?* Fat bombs are another popular topic and recipe in the keto community. When you first start keto, especially if you are coming out of a fat-free way of eating, it may be hard for you to eat fat in any shape, way or form. Fat bombs are designed to give you little blasts of fat in easy, sometimes fun, ways. You can make savory fat bombs with meats or fish, or you can make them sweet like candy. When I started keto, I immediately bought two fat-bomb cookbooks. Also, almost immediately, gave them away. I did this for two reasons: With the savory fat bombs, I found I would much rather just eat a plate of food for the same fat hit I was getting in something the size of a marble. With the sweet fat bombs, I quickly learned that I was no better off with keto candy than conventional candy. So, for me, no, I do not eat or even recommend fat bombs – but have at 'em if you like them (but be careful!).

- *Do I have to eat all the fat on my meat?* Well, the easiest way around this if you can't make yourself eat straight fat (not me, my friends: when people cut the fat off their steaks, I ask for it on my plate!) you can eat fattier cuts of meat that are marbled. If you are using ground beef, forget that love affair with "diet lean" which is usually 90% to 95% lean, and move to 80% or 85% lean. Enjoy salami, pepperoni, corned beef and pastrami. Enjoy bacon, duck, chicken (thighs and legs with skin on, please) and sausage. Buy the cheap cuts (usually fattier) and learn to slowly braise or use a slow cooker.

- *Do I have to add butter to my vegetables and oils to my salads?* Again, don't fear the fat. The answer to both is no, but do you really not like butter and oils? A lot of this is coming from the fat-free mindset that is so hard to shake. When you need to add some fat but don't want to go straight to butter or oil, try adding some sour cream. Make cream dressings with blue cheese or add full fat cheese to your salads, such as feta and brie.

- *What will happen if I am not hungry for three meals?* As odd as this question might seem, this is a source of anxiety and worry for a lot of people at the beginning, myself included. The natural progression of keto is that you are less often hungry because your hunger hormone (ghrelin) and fullness hormone (leptin) begin to throw off their shackles of insulin resistance. I was absolutely a three-meal-a-day plus two-snack-a day eater with plenty of after-dinner eating as well. The progression for me with keto started with having breakfast and coffee, then lunch and then something on the way home during my long commute. When I got home, I wasn't hungry, but I missed sitting down to dinner. I often ate when I wasn't hungry and that just didn't feel good. I thought to myself, if I want to eat dinner what is logical to cut out? I cut out lunches, but I hated that because I had a lunch hour at work. In the nice weather I could go for a walk, but in the colder weather I stayed in my office. I just didn't know what to do with myself for that hour, when I had always enjoyed shutting my door and having a leisurely lunch. I finally cut out breakfast (I had been a huge breakfast eater) but didn't want to forgo coffee. Then I moved to having a couple of coffees with heavy cream in the morning, a light lunch and then enjoyed a later dinner so that I would not look to eat in the evening and also, I would not be hungry in the morning.

  Another similar adjustment comes when you go out with friends to eat, and you are just not hungry. I know it is difficult in a social situation to not eat, especially if everyone is out to dinner or lunch at a restaurant. I would never say to eat anyway, especially if you have been trying so hard to get your hunger signals to where you can feel them. Have a cup of tea or coffee. If you are at about a 4 or 5 (on a scale of 1 to 10), it is okay to have something light. No one would question you if you just ordered a salad. The other thing is to plan to be hungry at the meal. If it is lunch, maybe have an earlier dinner the night before and cut your coffee or other beverage consumption in the morning. If it is dinner, that one is easy – perhaps have a light breakfast that day and then skip lunch or have something light but filling, like a few slices of salami and cheese.

  A lot of times this anxiety can come just from breaking your habits around food. If this is the situation, stop and breathe, and then ask yourself, "Am I hungry? What do I really need here?" I got very anxious at lunch, so in the nice weather I tried to get out for a walk, but eventually I adjusted my meals so that I was hungry at lunch. I would want to eat in the evenings after dinner, and in the midst of breaking that habit I would get very anxious. I stopped and asked myself what was really going on to cause that level of head hunger. Was I just unable to relax? What would help? Was I rethinking things that happened during the day that might have upset me? I realized they were only thoughts and I learned to sit with them and let the anxiety wash over and pass. Was it purely habit, for instance watching TV and eating? I would get up, brush my teeth and get ready for bed. Once you get used to not reacting to mealtimes, social situations, habits and anxiety, this question is moot. It won't even phase you that you are not eating the usual quantities and number of times.

- *What if I don't even know that I'm hungry?* If you have been strongly ruled by an external-locus-of-control way of eating (see CHAPTER 13, DANCING WITH LOW CARB AND KETO for further discussion on locus of control), you may have no clue what hunger is. This is because you relied on a clock or social situation to tell you it was time to eat. I do a lot of hunger-scale training with my clients (see Mindfulness Practice in CHAPTER 6 and also CHAPTER 12, THE HUNGER SCALE). In a nutshell, let me say that if you absolutely have no clue what feeling hungry is, try a short intermittent fast (see Appendix). If you must, have your coffee in the morning but go until dinner with nothing but water. Still not sure you are hungry? Wait until the next morning to eat. Short intermittent fasts clear up a lot of the "How do I know if I'm hungry?" questions. Another way to learn is to pay attention to how you feel after you eat. Please don't eat until the "I can't eat another bite" stage. Take one serving of whatever you are eating and put the fork down. Sit quietly and really home in on how you are feeling. Do you feel sort of neutral (5) – that you could probably eat a bit more without being stuffed? Okay – hold on to the feeling. Next time you wonder if you are hungry, recall this feeling you have right now. If this is how you feel you are not hungry enough to have a meal. CHAPTER 12, THE HUNGER SCALE gives you worksheets to practice this.

- *Do I have to get all the keto cookbooks and print all the recipes?* Not unless you are me. Seriously though, part of KISS (KEEP IT SIMPLE SWEETHEART, CHAPTER 14) is to do, or learn to do, keto with very simple ways of eating. Have some salami, cheese and olives at breakfast, or bacon and eggs if that's your jam. Have a salad with some protein, nuts, seeds and a nice dressing at lunch. Have a steak or roasted chicken with a cooked green vegetable on the side for dinner. Are you hungry during the day? Have some buttered bouillon or bone broth. Are you sorry you didn't have something for your commute home? Next time take some cheese wisps or string cheese, or olives or celery sticks to eat in the car. If you have a strict rule about not eating in the car, have something to eat before leaving work if you are really hungry and you have a long commute home. Truth be told, you can do successful keto on fast food if you have to. I wouldn't vouch for the quality of food, but in a pinch, I have had a McDonald's double cheeseburger, hold the bun and ketchup, add some mayo and extra pickle. No need to ever cook a thing if you don't want to. Once you have the bones of the program, then start branching out to new recipes. There are two caveats though: (1) Don't feel you ever have to have more complicated eating. But yet, (2) feel free to start tackling those interesting and complicated recipes from the start. You know what kind of personality you have, your time and your money constraints. You do not have to do anything one way or the other. Do what works for you, not anyone else on all the social media sites you visit.

- *Do I have to make only keto recipes?* Again, the answer is NO. Yes, you have to make recipes that are keto friendly, but you can take almost any recipe you have and convert it to a keto recipe. We make stuffed cabbage without rice in the stuffing. Adding well rung-out riced cauliflower or some chopped walnuts adds a nice texture for a recipe like this. We make loaded hamburgers, but don't use breadcrumbs. Serve them without the bun or you can make keto buns. We make a fantastic oven-baked fried chicken using, of all things, crushed BBQ pork rinds as the coating. We make macaroni and cheese but use tiny cauliflower florets instead of the pasta. Take whatever your favorite recipe is and be creative! Your recipes do not have to come out of a keto cookbook. If you want to make those purchases or do recipe downloads, that is up to you. You can approach this in a very simple manner just by getting creative with your own favorites.

- *What do I serve for dinner if I am the only one in the family doing keto?* This is a big question. When you first start, keep your meals simple such as roasted chicken, broiled fish, grilled burgers and steaks. Add for yourself and everyone else, a cooked green vegetable and a salad. The rest of the family can add potatoes, rice, pasta, bread or whatever they want. You can get very creative with family-friendly favorites and no one is the wiser. Read PART 5 – MEAL PLANNING AND SHOPPING. You will get a lot of solutions in that section.

- *How can I pack a lunch?* Okay, folks, there is more than one way to pack a lunch. Not everything revolves around sandwiches with bread. I write about this in CHAPTER 3 (STEP 1: ELIMINATE SUGAR AND BAKED GOODS) and again in CHAPTERS 15 AND 16 (LEARNING TO PLAN KETO MEALS AND LEARNING TO PLAN LOW CARB MEALS, respectively). Because this is among the things that most stumps people who are doing keto or low carb, I am putting it here again, so you read it more than once! Take a filling with you (deli meat, tuna salad, etc.), bring lettuce (not iceberg: it is too stiff), and make yourself rollups. (Side note: I have found from experience that any lettuce rollup made with a mayonnaise filling gets soggy in transit; bring the lettuce and filling separately and make your rollups when you are going to eat them.) "Can I have low carb (usually flour-based or corn-based) wraps?" NO, you cannot, if you are doing keto. Be creative. Use lettuce rollups or a cheese wrap or be even more creative and get out of the sandwich habit. "HUH? No sandwich for lunch?" Well, first of all, anything travels without bread. Use baggies and small containers and bring a fork. There are tons of grab-and-go foods too: Beef jerky, hard boiled eggs, salami and cheese (slices or rollups), cut veggies and ranch dip. Come on – you didn't become overweight by not understanding the concept of how to get food into your mouth!

- *Can I drink alcohol?* Yes, to a point. Mixed cocktail drinks are off the list because of the sugar content in mixers (and try not to get involved with "skinny-type" mixers – there may be too many chemicals and magic needed to make them taste like regular mixers). You can have one or two glasses of white wine or dry red wine. Note that the sweeter the wine, the higher the carbohydrate content. Straight spirits have no carbohydrates so yes, you can enjoy a whiskey, tequila or scotch or whatever. Just realize that your liver's primary job is to rid the body of toxins. While it is metabolizing the alcohol, you will not be burning fat. You may still be in ketosis because you are not consuming carbohydrates with the dry wine or spirits, but neither will you be burning fat at an optimal level. Some people have reported that they are much more sensitive to alcohol once they are on keto, so if you normally have more than one drink, stop at one and evaluate how you are feeling.

- *What if I'm traveling?* If you are traveling in a car this is very easy. It's your car (or a friend's car). Bring a cooler. All the grab-and-go foods I listed above travel well. Some don't even need the cooler! These foods are also very easy to restock from any store. Even most liquor stores now carry small vacuum packs of cheese and salami, sometimes even with olives! If you are traveling by plane, you can take food on the plane. Any bottled water or hot beverages like tea and coffee you can get once you are through the security gate. As a matter of fact, once you are through the security gate you can take any purchased beverages right on the plane with you. When I started keto, I would always ask for a fridge in my hotel room. I would stock it with what I had brought with me or find a little store near the hotel with keto-friendly foods. However, the longer I was keto, the more I realized I no longer needed to do this. I would have my coffee in the morning, and even a hotel breakfast of bacon and eggs and cheese. If I was hungry at lunch, I had no trouble finding keto-friendly foods and ditto at dinner. I usually enjoyed a meat-centric dinner like a nice ribeye and salad on the side. You will find that traveling on keto is actually easier than non-keto because you aren't hungry all the time and needing snacks when you get back to the hotel room. I have even thrown out doggie bags that I thought I would enjoy as an evening snack, but no longer wanted by the time I was ready to move on to the next adventure. This is even easier if you are following one of the steps of *Granny Keto Transitions Program*™ because you have fewer restrictions than you would have on keto. Aren't you glad you are learning to eat in a way that doesn't require weighing and measuring your food?

- *Is keto sustainable?* Yes and no. You must have a very strong reason to eat in a ketogenic manner, beyond the initial euphoria of weight loss, elimination of joint pain and a stomach that no longer complains. If you are someone who has reversed diabetes, eliminated non-alcoholic fatty liver disease or now finds herself finally pregnant due to the reversal of PCOS, then this way of eating can be sustainable for life. What is bread and pasta but flour and water? What is candy but sugar and coloring? What is junk food but junk? It becomes easy to give that up and never look back once your life has changed for the better. However, if you haven't seen those results yet, it can be very hard to make the commitment to stick with a ketogenic diet through carbohydrate withdrawal (known as "keto flu"), being the only person not partaking of burgers and fries at a restaurant or being the one person to say "no, thank you" to yumminess at parties and family gatherings. That does not mean that ketogenic eating is not sustainable. It means that your reasons for doing it might make adherence to this diet unsustainable. Although keto can be sustainable, you may feel that keto has run its course as you feel better and lose weight. In this case, it becomes an invaluable bridge to eating low carb, which is also an excellent means to attain weight loss and a healthy metabolism.

There are a few more questions that are more along the line of health concerns:

- *Will I become constipated?* One of the most common question is the worry about becoming constipated. You may find you will likely have regular, but less frequent and smaller bowel movements. This is because proteins can be easily broken down and absorbed in the intestines, so there is less output vs. a diet high in insoluble fiber. Your body just produces less waste because it is taking in less waste. Be sure to stay hydrated though.

- *Do I risk kidney damage?* There is strong research that disproves the common belief that eating protein above the recommended daily allowance damages kidney function. It was thought that excess protein causes kidney disease, but about 20 years ago that was disproven. If you have healthy kidneys, they will be able to handle the nitrogenous waste of protein. It is at stages 3 to 5 of kidney disease that you have to be concerned about too much protein. Protein itself will not cause kidney disease. Jason Fung uses a wonderful analogy using a sieve and blueberries, with the sieve being your kidneys and the blueberries being protein. If your sieve has no holes, it will hold the blueberries and the water will wash right over them and drain through the sieve. If you have holes in the netting, then the blueberries will fall through. It is not the blueberries that damage the sieve. It is the already-damaged sieve that is the problem. His books and the prominent study he refers to, are in the reference section of this book. I encourage you to listen to the short-lived "*Obesity Podcast*" with Jason Fung and Megan Ramos, hosted by Carl Franklin. In Episode 10 he specifically talks about the connection between protein and the kidneys.

- *Am I getting enough vitamins? Do I need supplements?* Some people may find a benefit from taking some electrolyte support (more fully discussed in CHAPTER 9, UNDERSTANDING KETO) like a magnesium or potassium supplement. A common worry is about getting enough vitamin C. This is not the case. The vitamin C present in meat and many vegetables, along with the vitamin C-sparing effect of low carb diets is enough to prevent scurvy, even without going out of your way to eat liver or other organ meat. The bottom line is that even on a diet of just muscle meat, you should expect to get enough vitamin C, along with all your other nutrients. Vitamin C seems to be of particular concern with the carnivore method (see Appendix) of keto, but there is no evidence to support that there will be a Vitamin C deficiency with this, or any other method of keto. The government RDA (recommended daily allowance) of Vitamin C and every other vitamin and mineral is determined by the high-glucose content of the Standard American Diet. Your needs for many of these vitamins and minerals are lower when you are on a well-formulated keto diet. This being said, you will want to work with your doctor to see what supplements your body requires, irrespective of eating keto.

GOOD TO KNOW...

Non-Alcoholic Fatty Liver Disease (NAFLD) is when too much fat builds up in liver cells. NAFLD, often reversible, is the most common liver disease in adults and children in Western countries. It is difficult to predict and often not detectable except for blood tests and imaging. It can, however, lead to impairment of the liver. NAFLD is also linked to an increased risk of other diseases, including heart disease, diabetes and kidney disease. It is caused by many factors including obesity, excess belly fat, insulin resistance, high intake of refined carbohydrates, sugary beverage consumption and impaired gut health. While you are working to correct these situations, let your liver "rest" and don't tax it by making it necessary to work to rid itself of fructose and alcohol.

PART FOUR
MAKE LOW CARB AND KETO YOUR LIFESTYLE

The legendary cellist Pablo Casals was asked why he continued to practice at age 90. "Because I think I'm making progress," he replied.

I think this quote beautifully sums up everything you are learning, especially in this section of *Breaking Free From Diet Prison: Common Sense Keto and Low Carb*.

Taking a page from Pablo Casals, making low carb and keto a lifestyle means practicing over and over and over again, those things that will make you successful along your journey.

This section presents three processes that, when practiced over and over again, will help you break free from diet prison and help you find peace with food. The first process is THE HUNGER SCALE, which will teach you to tune into your own body and allow you to decide for yourself when and what to eat, and not make eating decisions by a clock, a craving or a prescribed meal. Your hunger scale will teach you to trust when you are hungry and when you are satisfied enough to stop eating. It will take a lot of practice, but it starts with the first step.

The second process is learning to dance with your chosen lifestyle. Drawing on my 30 years of teaching dance and performance skills, I guide you to find the most successful ways to pull your eating out of the measuring, weighing and tracking hamster wheel of dieting. The skills in this chapter will free you to dance from your heart once and for all, and forever.

The third process is to KISS – KEEP IT SIMPLE SWEETHEART. Don't throw out the baby with the bathwater (throwing away all your progress because you had one misstep) or give up the minute something is harder than you thought it would be. Usually this is because *you* are making things harder than they need to be. You can start with something as simple as a Yes/No food list. Plan your meals around the "bones" of a food plan (PART 5, MEAL PLANNING AND SHOPPING). To start, if you need to, stay away from recipes with a lot of ingredients and directions. Eat simply and plainly. You must keep it simple when learning a new lifestyle. Practice simplicity over and over again.

Your success will lie in your ability to recognize that practice does not necessarily make perfect. What practice does is move you closer and closer to your goals!

Chapter Twelve

The Hunger Scale

In Chapter 6 (Step 4), I introduced the hunger scale in the mindfulness practice, along with the explanations and implications for each level of the scale. It is very important that you read and understand the narrative at each level of the hunger scale.

Learning to identify your level of hunger (or satiety) is one of the most important steppingstones to be successful in turning this whole process on its head and making the keto or low carb way of eating a lifestyle. Use the hunger scale (on paper or in your mind) every time you are questioning whether or not you are hungry and how hungry you are. When you have done it enough times particularly on paper, you will eventually be able to think about it before you reach for food. At this point, without much thought, I just stop for a second and put a number to my thought or urge to eat. Very often I will identify the number as being at or above 5 (satisfied to full) in which case my thoughts of food end right there. Other times I think about it further and ask myself what is causing me to want to eat even though my number is 5 or more. Oftentimes I can pinpoint the issue. It could be that I am bored, I had a disagreement with someone or that I am avoiding an activity. The next step is to not even think about the number but immediately recognize what is driving me and dismiss the hunger as head hunger or emotional hunger. Urges are addressed in Part 6, New Habits and Thoughts, but before you even begin to tackle that, learn to identify real hunger.

The other value in the hunger scale – other than sorting out head hunger from body hunger – is that, as you strive to learn to eat when hungry and stop when satisfied, you will find that if you are used to eating by the clock (lunchtime) or cues (smell those cookies) or triggers (anger, boredom, etc.) you really have never identified your hunger.

There are several ways to construct a scale. One that I like in addition to the one I present below, provides a visual. I remember at a Weight Watchers® meeting we all found red balloons on our chairs. We were asked to blow air into them until they started to take shape but weren't full. That represented what I call "5" on my scale: Neutral. On either side of that quantity of air were 1 to 4 and 6 to 10. It gave a great visual of your stomach being empty to totally full and ready to pop. Sometimes instead of visualizing the number I will see that red balloon in my mind's eye. I have also used a scale of 1 to 5, where 2 to 3 would sit at neutral, and full would be at 5. No matter what scale is comfortable for you, become aware of your hunger/fullness signals and where "neutral" lies for you.

GRANNY KETO'S HUNGER SCALE

1 - Ravenous and famished. You are starving, feeling faint or shaky.

2 - Really hungry. You may be preoccupied with food.

> **1–2: TRY NOT TO ALLOW YOURSELF TO GET HERE:** You will make poor food choices and eat too fast.

3 -Hungry. Ready for a meal but you don't feel like you need to stop everything and eat.

4 - Hungry. You could put off eating a bit longer. Distraction will take your mind off food, but not for long.

> **3–4: THIS IS A GOOD PLACE TO EAT:** You will be able to make good food choices and not wolf down your food.

5 - Neutral. If you are eating, you could stop here. Also, if you are not eating, your mind really doesn't go to food. You haven't hit 3 or 4 yet.

6 - Satisfied. A little more might make you full, but you could finish what you are eating and not be stuffed.

> **5–6: THIS IS A GOOD PLACE TO STOP EATING:** You have enjoyed your meal and can easily walk away from anything that is left. You will stop thinking about food or you might notice about 20 minutes after finishing that you are comfortably full.

7 - Full. You might start to feel a little uncomfortable and wish you didn't have those last few morsels.

8 - Very Full. At this point you are definitely feeling uncomfortable, and definitely wishing you hadn't continued eating.

> **7–8: STOP – REALLY:** You might find that you are determined to also have a dessert with a meal. I'm telling you now: You'll be sorry and please don't!

9 - Overfull, stuffed, uncomfortable, bloated, stomachache.

10 -Absolutely stuffed. You are not only uncomfortable, but you may be nauseous, sweating, need to sleep and painfully full.

> **9–10: FORGIVE YOURSELF.** Then, if you can, get up and walk around. Don't make it worse by beating yourself up and punishing yourself by eating even more. If you find yourself here often then it is time to talk with a counselor or do some serious work and introspection. You are getting here not because the food tastes too good to stop. There are other, deeper issues, and I implore you to work on figuring them out.

You will notice levels 9 and 10 include the narrative: "Forgive and learn the lesson." You can never do good things for yourself if you are coming from a place of hating yourself. What can you learn and what can you do about what you have learned? I have been dieting for 55 years now. I have finally forgiven myself and have learned my lessons.

A Hunger Scale for You to Use

Tune in to your level of hunger/fullness using this scale.

1 - Ravenous and famished. I may be starving, feeling faint or shaky.

2 - Really hungry. I may be preoccupied with food.

3 -Hungry. Ready for a meal but I don't feel like I need to stop everything and eat.

4 - Hungry. I could put off eating a bit longer. Distraction will take my mind off food, but not for long.

5 - Neutral. I'm eating and I could stop here – OR – I haven't eaten yet and I could take it or leave it.

6 - Satisfied. A little more might make me full, but I could finish what I am eating and not be stuffed.

7 - Full. I'm starting to feel a little uncomfortable and wish I didn't have those last few morsels.

8 - Very Full. At this point I'm definitely feeling uncomfortable, and I'm definitely wishing I hadn't continued eating.

9 - Overfull, stuffed, uncomfortable, bloated, stomachache.

10 -Absolutely stuffed. I'm not only uncomfortable, but I'm nauseous, sweating, need to sleep, and painfully full.

What are the Lessons I Have Learned?

Before we leave working with your hunger scale, there is something to address, and that is whether or not you should ever eat if you are not hungry. I counsel my clients that is okay to eat even if they are not hungry, but we explore that before they go off on their way saying, "Miriam said I could eat even if I'm stuffed." I am not saying that at all. What I am saying is that food and meal-taking is entrenched in our cultures. There is food at happy occasions, such as weddings and birth celebrations. There is food at holidays, such as Thanksgiving and Christmas. There is food at sad occasions, such as funerals. There is food to show love, such as the special dinner or dessert requested by the birthday person. Like it or not, food does show love. The problem arises when the food itself becomes love and happiness and when the association of food to sadness develops at a visceral level for us.

Now when we are upset, we eat; when we are lonely, we eat; when we are happy, we eat. There is also that "short-chain" reaction, i.e., "My boss yelled at me so I'm going to eat cupcakes." These circumstances do not give you permission to eat when you are not hungry.

Do not give in to food pushers. "Here, I made your favorite pie, and you will hurt my feelings if you don't eat it" or "Take one more bite, it won't kill you." Furthermore, if you ate lunch which you brought with you and the office orders out, you shouldn't have a second lunch or eat food because it is there, or it is free.

However, you do not have to be at a 5 or less on the scale to eat. Maybe you had a late and satisfying breakfast and intend to skip lunch but there is a mid-day Christmas party at the office and there is a favorite dessert you like. You can wrap it up for later, or you can have a bite or piece and enjoy it. You do not then have to hate yourself because the food was off your plan or you ate when you were already at a 6. Have it, enjoy it and move on. Don't make yourself sick at a Thanksgiving dinner. Let's say you did have too many appetizers because you were talking with friends and were not paying attention. Before you know it, you are already at a 5 or 6. To handle this, go back to the Good-Better-Best model introduced in CHAPTER 5. GOOD would be to make a plate and have it but at least don't have seconds or desserts. BETTER would be to take a little of your most favorite thing and just eat that. BEST would be to not eat. If it is at a family member's house, you can ask to wrap up a plate to go. The point is, eating when you are not hungry does not have to be black or white, right or wrong. You can look at Good-Better-Best and take the route that is best for you. Don't let GOOD derail you because it is not BEST. GOOD is a valid option on the journey.

Another situation would be if you are going out to dinner, but you had a late and satisfying breakfast. Let yourself get a little hungry during the day – have a snack or half of your lunch, so that you are at a 5 or below when you go out to dinner. But if you are not that hungry, you don't have to sit there and drink a glass of water while everyone else is eating. Have just an appetizer or salad. Join the meal and don't feel guilty.

Eating past a 6 or 7 is not a moral issue. It is not the tipping point between whether you are a good person or a bad person, a worthy person or an unworthy person. It is a question of how do you want to feel? There is the physical layer. You certainly don't want to make yourself sick or feel so bad you are popping TUMS all night. The mental layer is actually more important. How will you feel if you eat food not on your plan and feel way past full? Can you give yourself permission or will you beat yourself up, hate yourself and maybe get totally derailed from your food plan? It is important to see yourself through several of these situations. Sometimes eat, sometimes don't eat. Eventually you will learn what is best for you. One size does not fit all!

GOOD TO KNOW...

Wrangling with your hunger scale can often be just wrangling with head hunger ("It's lunchtime so I'm hungry for lunch"), heart hunger ("I'm lonely and food always makes me feel better") or habit ("I always pick up and eat a croissant when I pass this bakery"). However, there is very much a hormonal biological basis for when you feel true hunger. Leptin and ghrelin, known as the "hunger hormones" along with insulin, all play important roles in hunger regulation. Ghrelin, produced by the stomach, is responsible for feelings of hunger. Leptin, produced by the fat cells in your body, send a signal of fullness. Unfortunately, when someone is obese, that individual will have too much leptin in the blood, causing a lack of sensitivity to the hormone. A condition known as leptin resistance occurs. That is why you can eat and never feel full, making it hard to find the "satisfied" mark on your hunger scale. That does not mean that you need to give up. Your body will begin to self-regulate if you exercise portion control and eat few, if any, foods that keep you hungry like carbohydrates that raise your insulin levels.

Chapter Thirteen

Dancing with Low Carb and Keto

Imagine being 70 years old and saying to yourself "Time to enter my food in my tracker." Really? Okay, you might not be 70 years old now, but why use a method of weight loss that you won't want to continue for the rest of your life? This is the overall problem with any diet. You are on OR you are off! Even diets that claim to be a lifestyle, like Weight Watchers, still involve counting and tracking in order to stay on the straight and narrow. Chances are that if you are a life-long dieter you come to this fork in the road. You can keep on counting and tracking or choose the road that finally gives you some freedom and peace with such a basic need as fueling your body. What is interesting is that with many diets you can follow either road. The choice is really yours.

You may have heard of the term, *locus of control*. This refers to the degree to which people believe that they have control over the outcome of events in their lives as opposed to external forces beyond their control. This is the root of choosing a fear-based path over a freedom-based path. After so many years of failed dieting, you may have come to believe that you have to be told what to eat, when to eat and how much to eat. You may hear yourself saying:

"I can't trust myself to know how much to eat."

"I need to be punished for overeating, bingeing and being too stupid to follow a diet."

"If I eat one cookie, I will finish the bag, so I either need to not have them at all or count them out very carefully."

"Other people are smarter than I am."

"I have never been successful and there is no reason to think I will be now."

"And for all of this, I need to be told what to eat and how much."

Here you have an external locus of control. You believe that you cannot make decisions about what, when, how much and how to eat because past experience has left you in a state of feeling like a failure when relying on your own decisions.

The freedom path means that you learn to trust your body. You learn to trust what foods give you energy and make you feel well. You learn what foods fuel you and what foods sap you. You learn to sit with feelings that previously sent you to find food as a buffer so that you would not feel or face these feelings. You become comfortable with the discomfort because you know that feelings cannot kill you and that they will pass. You will not need to use food to avoid them. You learn to have joy in your life and learn to fill your life with experiences instead of using food to fill your life.

The freedom path may be much harder in the short run than the fear path, because you have so much learning to do – about foods, about quantities that make you feel best, about hunger signals and about yourself. Once you have allowed yourself the feeling of "Maybe, just maybe, I can trust myself to do this and be responsible for the success I will have," you have crossed over to an internal locus of control. You build it like a muscle, one success building upon the next. But you have to at least start. I want you to build those muscles and dance down the road of the freedom path.

I was a successful belly dance teacher and performer for over 30 years. My dancers were well-known throughout New England. Any musician could spot a student of Amira Jamal (my professional dance name) because those dancers were able to dance, without choreography, to any music played for them. More importantly, they danced from the heart. You will see that the lessons I learned as a dance teacher and performer can be applied to any way you choose to eat along any of the steps of *Granny Keto Transitions Program*™ or with any program you are following.

TRUST YOURSELF

Here is the story of one of my dancers, Julia. She is talented and a hard worker, and I felt incredibly lucky to have her as a student. For her first recital with me she had worked very hard on a piece of choreography. During the dress rehearsal she asked several times to stop the music so she could consult her notes. Finally, I said, "Julia, give me your choreography notes. Maybe I can help you." I took the sheet of paper from her and ripped it in half. Julia – and the rest of the class – were stunned. It looked as though she was going to cry. I said, "NOW you dance. Dance from your heart." Did I know for sure that Julia would do a beautiful performance? Did I know she would survive? Yes, and Yes. But how did I know this? I knew this because she knew the steps and the combinations and how to move to the music. I knew that Julia knew it all and could trust herself to dance from her heart.

What does this have to do with eating low carb and keto? Everything! **Low Carb and Keto Lesson:** You do not have to weigh, measure, count or track your food in order to be successful. However, you do need to be informed and mindful, and you need to trust yourself. Just as with dancing, where you need to know steps, combinations, nuances and how one thing works with the music and another thing does not, you can't just "eat low carb" or just "eat keto" without an understanding of what it is you are eating. You need to start by learning the steps. These steps are made from the knowledge and understanding of where your carbs come from and how much each food "costs" you. With keto, these steps are made from understanding your macronutrients and how they will put you into ketosis and ultimately help you lose weight. With low carb, these steps are made from your understanding of carbohydrates and your decision about what foods you want to include in your eating plan.

At the very least, if you eat from the Yes/No food list (CHAPTER 10, WAYS OF DOING KETO), you will only need to track your carbohydrates to make sure you do not go over your total allowance if you are doing keto. If you are aiming for a low carb lifestyle, eat from the same Yes/No food list but keep foods such as baked goods, grains, legumes, fruit or foods containing sugar to only one or two servings a day. With regard to keto, keep in mind that you can still eat keto by following the Yes/No list, but please know that keto is not necessarily a weight loss diet. It can be, but at the start you may need to be stricter than just tracking carbohydrates. This may mean paying close attention to foods such as dairy, nuts and seeds. If you track only carbohydrates and keep them to a total of 20, you will most likely lose weight at the beginning, but your weight loss may stall even though your innards are continuing to get healthy. Your fasting insulin and blood sugars will go down, your lipid profile will improve, and your blood pressure will normalize. You also may "shape shift," meaning that you might not lose any weight but might go down a size or two in clothing. This is because your body composition will be changing. However, if you eat when you are not hungry or you eat when you are beyond full, it will simply be too much food for your body to process. The quality of the food will make you healthier, but the quantity of food might keep you fat!

If you have dieted your whole life, your safe way to approach low carb or keto is to weigh, measure and track your food, because, as usual, an external source is telling you when you have had enough. However, you can lose weight without doing any of those things. If you are willing to put in some work and listen to your body and eat only when hungry and stop when satisfied (see CHAPTER 12, THE HUNGER SCALE) you might not lose weight quickly, but it will become a comfortable lifestyle and the weight loss will be lasting. You will ultimately achieve goals that you set for yourself. Tracking the elements of your intake (macros and calories) is on one end of the process and going totally "freestyle" is on the other. Your success may lie somewhere in between.

THE MINDSET AND PAYING ATTENTION

Let's look at the concept of "as if" for dancing – or anything in life. Walk as if you have confidence and you will. Smile as if you have confidence and you will. Dance as if you have confidence and you will. Exude pride as if you have it and you will. **Low Carb and Keto Lesson:** Stop telling yourself you can't do it. With every meal you prepare and with every bite you take, tell yourself "I am smart and intelligent, and I can do this. I am eating low carb (or keto) and every step of the way I am moving toward better health and achieving my goals." Keep it up and you will move towards better health and achieving your goals. *First you have to believe.* Why do I make this the first step before even starting the road to making low carb and keto a lifestyle? I do this because you need to know that you are worthy and capable of making this change in your life. I do this because you need to know you are intelligent enough to do it and to make decisions about the food that is in front of you. I found for myself that just learning about getting into that correct mind-space was more valuable than any practical aspects of learning keto and low carb.

From there, when I was teaching my dancers to dance from the heart, we spent time listening to all sorts of music and seeing how the music made our bodies move. **Low Carb and Keto Lesson:** Does a food make you feel good, give you energy and satisfy you, or does some food make you feel nauseous, uncomfortable, tired and leave you wanting more while sending you into a binge? Your next step in learning to dance is by noticing how food makes you feel. You may have food sensitivities that you never noticed because your default physical feeling is crummy. Sometimes you aren't even aware of this because you are so accustomed to feeling sub par. So many people in the low carb and keto communities remark that they never knew they could feel so much better by cutting out something like dairy or eggs. Sometimes eliminating just one food can even end the binges because you are satisfied with what you are eating and are not searching for a way to feel better. Start paying attention to what you are eating. You are wiser than you think. Do you feel bloated after a meal? What was in it? Do you need a nap after lunch? What did you eat? Are you itchy? What caused that itchiness (for me it was eggs - who knew?)? Are you sneezing? Is your throat scratchy? Do you just feel sapped of energy? What have you eaten since breakfast? Pay attention! Become your own detective.

LEARNING THE STEPS

Next comes learning the steps. Not just learning but practicing – over and over again! My dancers kept notebooks with the steps we were learning. Every class started with drills. It didn't matter if you were a new student or had studied with me for ten or more years. We drilled the same steps every week and slowly added new ones to our notebooks. **Low Carb and Keto Lesson:** This is where you keep your own notebook with steps. Even with a Yes/No list you still need to know counts (carbs, specifically) in order to be successful with weight loss. List your favorite foods and what a good portion would be. You can do this by putting foods into a food calculator like My Fitness Pal or Carb Manager and then writing down the protein, fat and carbohydrate count in each unit of food. You can use a book like *Dr. Atkins NEW Carbohydrate Gram Counter* by Robert Atkins. I found this easy to carry with me when I would not be preparing my own meals at my own house. Mindfulness with this approach to eating low carb and keto is more than half the battle.

I quickly learned that carbohydrates in vegetables add up, that something like canned tuna fish is high in protein and that I was not eating nearly enough fat. Even if you do the Dancing with Low Carb and Keto method, it is still important to understand the macros (steps) you should aim for when eating keto, specifically: 20 carbohydrates total, net or combined (see CHAPTER 10, WAYS OF DOING KETO). When you eat keto your carbohydrate intake will come to about 5% of your caloric intake, with the rest of your calories making up about 20% protein and 75% fat. These macros can be different for each person. Some people are especially sensitive to carbohydrates and cut back even further, while others may find that they can process more protein or a few more carbohydrates. The point here is to listen to your body and decide what makes it sing and dance! With regard to eating low carb, you will have to find your own answer. For example, does bread make you feel hungry or do foods that contain wheat make you feel unwell?

The food restrictions, especially on keto, are less than what people generally think. Look at the number of keto cookbooks that are available to you. Just about the only ingredients that you do not use are caloric sugars and any products coming from wheat, grains or legumes (for instance, flour or corn starch). There are substitutions for it all, and there are many creative and talented recipe developers. One person whom I interviewed on my podcast has even come up with a yeast bread. She makes breads, dinner rolls, hamburger rolls, etc. with this recipe. You are only as limited as your mind tells you that you are.

A meaningful quote for me and many of my clients, and which I have quoted several times throughout this book is: *Whatever you do, never run back to what broke you.* This means that you need to be aware of whether it is the concept of a food that triggers your eating behavior or whether it is the ingredients. For some, it is sugar and flour themselves that trigger eating behaviors. By eliminating those foods, people can travel on their low carb and keto journeys enjoying sugar-free cookies and candy, or wheat-free breads and pastas, etc. For me, personally, it is the concept of the food that triggers my eating behavior. One sugar-free cookie might as well be 10. A slice of wheat-free bread might as well be a whole loaf. Know yourself. If food concepts do not trigger you, then you will probably feel the low carb and keto "pinch" very little.

PUTTING STEPS TO MUSIC

Although I did not teach choreography as a rule, I would start my beginner dancers with two or three very simple dances so that they could practice which steps went with which music. They learned quickly what steps matched which music so they could make up routines for themselves. Better yet, they were never puzzled when faced with live music that in no way resembled the recorded music to which they had practiced, even if it was the same song. **Low Carb and Keto Lesson:** Once you have practiced your steps and have also practiced your mindset and food feedback (i.e., foods that feel good in your body and quantities that work), it is pretty easy to tell if something fits your needs or not. Take your basic foods that you like and especially those that are easy to pack if you need to bring food to work. Don't make it complicated. At the beginning, weigh and measure everything and learn what a portion size is and how much protein, fat and carbohydrate is in that serving. (To start with, just make sure you track your carbohydrates and keep them within a 20 total, net or combined carb limit.) If you are not new to dieting, you may know already how to figure portion sizes without weighing or measuring. The picture on the next page is a visual that might help. I have had several clients who are successful just using the visual and never use a measuring spoon, a measuring cup or a food scale.

PORTION SIZE

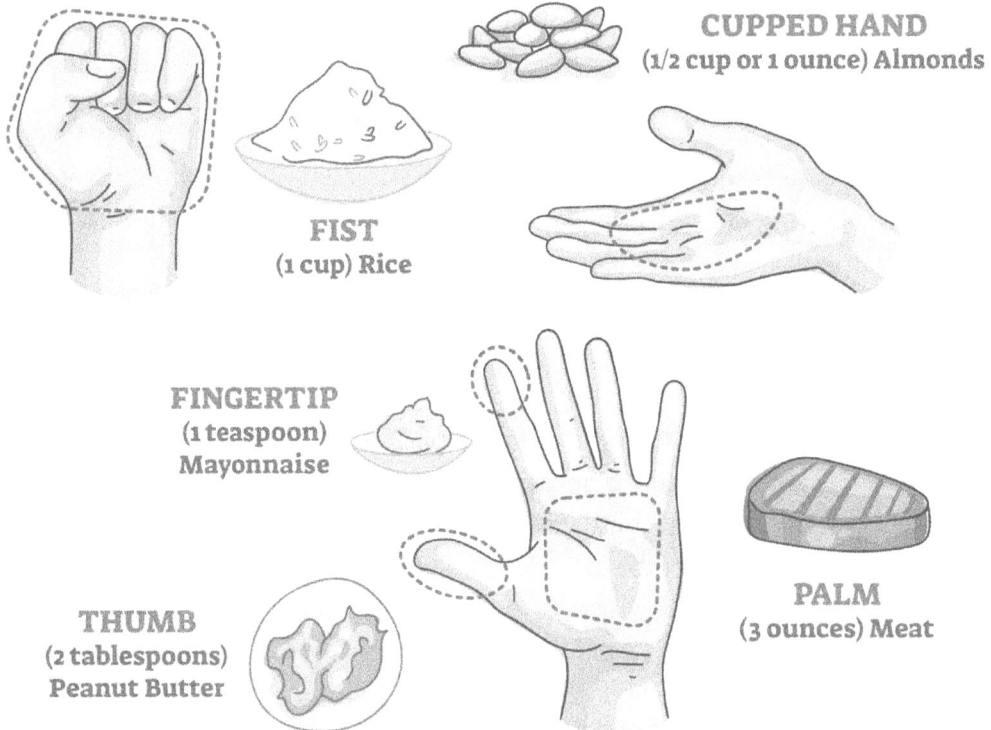

CUPPED HAND
(1/2 cup or 1 ounce) Almonds

FIST
(1 cup) Rice

FINGERTIP
(1 teaspoon)
Mayonnaise

THUMB
(2 tablespoons)
Peanut Butter

PALM
(3 ounces) Meat

Going back to your list of "steps", look at the macros for the following examples using keto-based requirements. (If eating low carb, the same ideas hold, although you might be eating a bit more carbohydrate and somewhat less fat.)

- 3 ounces of tuna fish canned in water: Total carbs: 0 (great!); Protein: 20; Fat: 2.5 (that's nothing! You will have to add mayonnaise to this lunch or treat yourself to tuna packed in olive oil!).

- 3 ounces of hamburger (85/15): Total carbs: 0 (great!); Protein: 19; Fat: 22 (much better!).

- 3 ounces of fried pork belly (if you like bacon and have not tried this, get some!): Total carbs: 0 (great!); Protein: 11 (you could use a little bit more); Fat: 21 (great!). (The pork belly has a great fat to protein ratio, but it's not a food you need to eat. Even though people are gaga over bacon on keto, you do not have to eat bacon or any pork product on keto (see Chapter 11, Questions and Dispelling Myths).

By knowing the steps of the dance (i.e., macros of the foods) you can eventually start to put together meals which will not require measuring and tracking. You will learn when some mayonnaise or butter will round out your daily macros, whether a salad will add a few safe carbs or whether you haven't had enough protein and you might want to add a sprinkling of cheese to your meal. **You are starting to dance to the music!** Create a few meals that you can rotate and stick with for the first few weeks.

- Breakfasts could be scrambled eggs and bacon or (my favorite) Caprese salad, which is mozzarella, fresh tomatoes, fresh basil, olive oil and a sprinkling of balsamic vinegar. For low carb feel free to add some toast.

- Lunches could be salad. If you make your own and are following keto, weigh, measure and track it the first few times. Vegetables pack a lot of carbs and you need to be mindful of this. Add some feta cheese and hard-boiled eggs or tuna with mayonnaise and crunchy, diced vegetables (celery and bell pepper). For low carb, you may want to add high-carb vegetables like carrots or cherry tomatoes or a piece of fruit.

- Keep dinner simple. Have steak or chicken thighs with a cooked vegetable like asparagus or broccoli. For low carb, if you haven't been eating many other carbohydrate-rich foods during the day, you may add a portion of potatoes, pasta or rice.

Again, these are your steps, the steps you have decided to learn and put to the music. Practice them over and over again. When I started keto, I would weigh and measure, and then after a few times "eyeball" the portion but then weigh and measure to see how spot on I was. Eventually I would just make myself a plate and be done with it! My foods fit my macro goals just as my dance steps fit the music. Identify your favorite low carb and keto foods. Then design your plate so you can be sure that you are eating a healthy and satisfying way at every meal – enough fats, adequate protein and the best carbohydrate choices.

Branching Out into More Complicated Steps and Music

After my dancers learn simple steps with simple music we branch out into more complicated steps and more complicated music. But again, it doesn't happen without practice. It does become easier once the dancer understands the concepts and the nuances of the steps or hears the music in a more educated way so that the complicated and nuanced movements flow with the music. **Low Carb and Keto Lesson:** If you become tired of basic meals and foods it is time to branch out into recipes. But don't rush this. You must learn the basic steps before you can start to put together combinations via recipes. If the recipe does not already have nutritional information, it is a good idea to work with some sort of recipe builder (or write everything out by hand) so that you are aware of the macro counts. Once you have followed a recipe and you understand the ingredients and portions you can begin to do it on your own (very advanced non-choreography).

Baking is a science, so it is important to precisely follow the recipe. However, once you have made something like a soup or a stir-fry, you can alter the flavor profiles or quantities of ingredients while still having a sense of the macro count.

Find recipes that the whole family will love. Sort out flavor profiles so that you become comfortable changing up recipes as you need to. By flavor profiles I mean that you can take a pound of hamburger and season it with Italian seasonings one night, TexMex another and Asian another. Change up the veggies or side dishes. If you are eating low carb and know how the recipe generally fits into your food plan, you can add diced potatoes one night and pasta the next. You do not have to rework the entire recipe to dance with it!

One word about not being exact on all the counts: Some people are extremely sensitive to carbohydrates. For instance, you may have very severe insulin resistance, type 2 diabetes or non-alcoholic fatty liver disease. You may have yo-yo dieted your whole life so that your metabolism is wonky. In these instances, you may find that you don't have as much leeway as I am suggesting here. However, even when you are varying recipes you can begin to trust yourself. With straight-away foods – like an egg or a slice of cheese, or a recipe that you always make the same way, it is even easier.

This and Not Also That

A dancer must also understand the concept of "this and not also that." A dancer must understand not to make her dancing too busy. She has to learn not to dash from one end of the stage to the other, to twirl her hands around incessantly or repeat the same steps over and over again. **Low Carb and Keto Lesson:** In order to stay within your macros for the day without the counting, you have to make sure that your eating day is not too busy. As I said earlier, especially with keto, eating this way is for health, not necessarily weight loss. But if you do want to lose weight there are certain things you have to adhere to whether eating low carb or keto. The first rule is no grazing! If you are eating enough fat, you will immediately be able to stick with three meals a day with no physical need to snack (breaking a snack habit is another story). When you first start and you aren't used to eating so much fat, you might need a snack because your meals might not hold you, but in no way should you graze. That means no hands full of nuts, no grabbing some salami or cheese from the fridge and no munching on baby carrots all day long.

In terms of a day being busy, I mean more than just grazing. If you have had a green smoothie for breakfast, go light on the salad at lunch or cooked vegetables at dinner so you have more room for protein and fat. If you have had seafood (which packs a punch in the protein department) for a meal, try to make one of your other meals a little lighter on protein – such as just having a piece of cheese or a couple of hard-boiled eggs. Do not worry about too much protein (very little chance that you are eating too much) but do try not to have a 12-ounce rib-eye steak for each meal – not that you would, but I hope you get my point. It is fine to look at your food meal by meal and indeed I recommend that, but try also to look at your day as a whole in addition to meal by meal. A good place to start is look at your plate and ask yourself, "Will this get me to my goal?" Food by food (step-by-step) and plate by plate (combination-by-combination), you will find yourself dancing in no time!

Even though a low carb lifestyle is less strict than keto, you still need to make sure that you are not overloading your plate with the same food meal after meal or eating the same foods all the time. Did you have toast at breakfast? Maybe in that case use your carbohydrates at lunch in a rice bowl. Did you have rice at lunch? Maybe in that case have a higher-carb vegetable at dinner such as carrots or beets. Your body will thank you for not eating the same foods over and over again at every meal.

Some people meal plan so that dinner on Monday would be the perfect lunch on Tuesday to complement breakfast and dinner that day. Change up leftovers by varying the side vegetables or the dressing on your salad. Eventually you will not even need the guidance of meal planning. It's just dancing!

NON-NEGOTIABLES

With dancing there are non-negotiables. A frown and a down-turned head could erase months and months of work and dull the beauty that the dancer worked so hard to achieve for her performance level. **Low Carb and Keto Lesson:** There are some specific non-negotiables. Let me start with keto. These non-negotiables would be no grains (not even oatmeal for breakfast), no starchy vegetables (that's right – throw out your bags of baby carrots), no fruit (except berries after you have had keto success for a while) and no refined carbohydrates, legumes or starchy vegetables.

It is harder to define "non-negotiables" for a low carb lifestyle because if you are allowing all foods in moderation, what is there to omit? However, you can decide for yourself how to define your low carb lifestyle. If you are following *Granny Keto Transitions Program*™, Steps 1 and 2 for instance, you may have your own list of non-negotiables such as no sugar or foods containing sugar, no baked goods, no grains or legumes. On Step 3, you might allow yourself a dessert once in a while but say no potatoes or bread. The point is, this is *your* lifestyle, *your* decisions and *your* dance.

BUILD YOUR OWN ROAD

It is admittedly difficult when all your life you have dieted and have followed someone else's rules. Think of this experience, this dancing, as building your own road with your own parameters and boundaries. With practice and experience you will eventually find the way to hold up your head and smile. You will dance confidently and avoid all the stumbling blocks of the past while embracing the non-negotiables of the present. You will learn how to dance from the heart, I promise.

The trick is to be mindful. When you use a digital tracker or track by hand, you get to the end of the day and an outside source (the tracker) tells you when you have had enough to eat for the day. Once you learn to dance from the heart and make a commitment to the non-negotiables, you will find that low carb, keto or any step along *Granny Keto Transitions Program*™, is actually a very easy way of eating. Remember: you want to establish an internal locus of control and weaken the external one. You might be tempted to go running back to the external controls (weighing, measuring, tracking) if you have had an eating "frenzy," no matter how long or short, large or small. Don't do that. Just start with the very next meal. Dance!

Notice I say DO it again not try it again. Trying connotes a certain lack of commitment. "Oh, I'll try this out and see how I like it or if it works out." NO – consider this a commitment, a DO. And remember, nothing and no one will be perfect from the start. Give yourself that grace. Don't give up too soon. Don't just try it out. Do it and do it over and over again until it becomes right for you. This is practicing. THIS is freedom.

One last word about choosing internal control vs. external control or freedom vs. fear. Don't misunderstand what the freedom path is. It is not permission to eat anything you want, as much of it as you want and any time you want. The true freedom path, the true dancing, is to make the right decisions for yourself, grocery shopping excursion after grocery shopping excursion, recipe after recipe and meal after meal. It is work. But, as you do it over and over again it becomes easier and easier because you are not tiring out your decision-making muscles with all the heavy lifting that comes with learning new things.

GOOD TO KNOW...

"Act as if" has research support as a behavioral intervention. Behavioral interventions work to change people's lives from an outside-in approach. By altering one's external circumstances (acting "as if"), we can change the ways we think and feel about ourselves. Very often we engage in "self-sabotage" and we act ineffectively despite knowing better ways of handling difficult situations, mostly because of our automatic thoughts. Acting "as if" can help alter these dysfunctional thoughts, even when we truly believe them. Our body and psyche hate cognitive dissonance. This means that your body and your mind strive to bring thoughts and actions into alignment. Eventually, visualizing what we want to do and how we want to be will bring our ultimate actions into alignment with those thoughts.

Chapter Fourteen

K.I.S.S. - Keep It Simple Sweetheart

Do you have the dancing part down? Do you understand the terms internal locus of control and external locus of control? Do you understand the difference between the fear path and the freedom path choices of eating? Great! Now let's put dancing into practice with KISS: Keep it Simple Sweetheart.

In my "Ask Granny" feature on my former website, I have had so many people ask me the following questions with regard to keto: Do I have to eat anything made with coconut? Do I have to eat bacon? Do I have to drink coffee with a lot of fat in it? What if I don't like coffee at all? What if I don't like cream in my tea? Do I have to fast? Do I have to eat organic? Is keto expensive? Do I have to weigh and measure? Do I have to track and count macros? Do I have to eat fat bombs? Do I have to eat all the fat on meat? Do I have to add butter to my vegetables? With both low carb and keto, I have gotten these sorts of questions: Do I have to count calories? What will happen if I am not hungry for three meals? What if I don't even know when I'm hungry? Do I have to get keto and low carb cookbooks? Do I have to make only keto and low carb recipes? What do I serve for dinner if I am the only one eating this way? How can I pack a lunch? Can I drink alcohol? What if I am traveling? (The answers to these, and more, questions are in CHAPTER 11, QUESTIONS AND DISPELLING MYTHS.)

Okay, you are all making this way more complicated than it has to be! Let's take dancing again. There is the goofy way of dancing in your living room and then there are the professional ballroom dancers. Oh my, do you think there is anything in between? I'm not even going to give you the answer to that because I think you know it! Eating keto, low carb or any one of the steps of *Granny Keto Transitions Program*™ can be placed along that same spectrum. Somewhere in between is where most of us find success with this way of eating. It doesn't have to be an absolute choice between "Lazy Keto" (see Appendix) or weighing, measuring and tracking every morsel of food that goes into your mouth. It doesn't have to be an absolute choice between eating catch-as-catch-can or planning out every single bite you will eat between now and next week. It doesn't have to be an absolute choice between eating plain dull foods day after day or remodeling your kitchen, buying every cooking gadget known to man and cooking only from fancy cookbooks and recipe blogs.

I once had a girlfriend say to me, "I could do keto if I had someone to shop and cook for me." First of all, this is a helpless and needless way to look at things. Second of all, it is a window into the fact that a lot of people think that keto (or any of the TRANSITIONS steps) is a lot more complicated than it is. You do not need special kitchen equipment or special cookbooks or spices or dishes.

You do not need a pocketful of money to buy only organic produce and grass-fed or pasture-raised meats (another huge myth!). You do not need hours to make meal plans, grocery shop and prepare meals. You don't. You really don't.

The best way to start with keto or any of the steps in TRANSITIONS is to keep things simple. Please remember K.I.S.S. Keep It Simple Sweetheart. I repeat: Eating this way does not have to be complicated. Don't make it so.

In addition, if you have been eating mostly processed and catch-as-catch-can foods up to now, you don't have to make a huge leap into being able to eat keto especially if your finances are an issue. There is nothing wrong with starting keto with baloney, hot dogs, canned fish, frozen vegetables, lots of eggs and sliced cheese. Your first and only commitment to keto needs to be to keep your carbs low. Yes, you do want to look for seasonings and spice mixes that do not contain sugar or things like corn or potato starch. This is where, even keeping it simple it might be a good idea to check recipes so that you can make some of these in your own kitchen! Most mustards don't have carbs and there are plenty of sugar-free BBQ sauces and ketchups to choose from. Check your processed meats for those same ingredients (sugar, corn or potato starch, high-fructose corn syrup, etc.) but with a little bit of label sleuthing you can start out with this familiar way to eat, eventually moving to more natural and healthier foods. In this community there are people known as the "Keto Police" or "Keto Snobs" – listen only to kind advice and not to them. You do keto and low carb your way as best you can. Anything moving towards a healthy lifestyle is an improvement. Keep it simple. When you are ready to move on, you will.

I am going to say a word here about cooking for, and eating with, non-keto and non-low carb family and friends. This is truly a soap-box moment so please indulge me. I understand (and encourage you) if you do need some support from your family and friends. However, this is *your* journey. You cannot expect them to never have another snack, piece of bread, potato, pasta or cookie. Don't whine you cannot do this because you do not have support. Hopefully at the very least, they would not tempt you with the "off plan" foods they are eating, and not make fun of you for trying something new. You can do your part to find "friendly" keto and low carb recipes. For instance, I make a popular macaroni and cheese with cauliflower, and I also make a wonderful keto cheesecake.

If your reasons are strong enough for finding a new eating lifestyle, THEN YOU CAN BE STRONG ENOUGH TO FIND A WAY. Stop trying and just do it. It's *your* why and *your* journey. Have your own back and don't think you can't do it without support. Remember to KISS!! Don't make separate meals for family members. Find a way to keep it simple but add things for other family members (see the dinner worksheets for LEARNING TO PLAN KETO MEALS AND LEARNING TO PLAN LOW CARB MEALS IN CHAPTERS 15 and 16, respectively). You can keep this simple even while pleasing everyone in your family. Trust me on this!

Good to Know...

There is scientific evidence that you will succeed best on *Granny Keto Transitions Program*™ and also with keto if you take my advice and keep it simple! An Indiana University study compared dieting behavior of women following two radically different diet plans and found that the more complicated people thought their diet plan was, the sooner they were likely to drop it. Even if you believe you can succeed, thinking that the diet is complex can undermine efforts. The more like rocket science one's diet plan feels, the less likely that one will succeed with long-term adherence and maintenance.

Part Five
Meal Planning and Shopping

- Learning To Plan Keto Meals
- Learning To Plan Low Carb Meals
- Protocol Meal Planning
- Grocery Shopping

In Parts 5 and 6, I will give you lessons and worksheets that will help you on your journey. I may repeat the text you already read in other chapters or ask you to go back and reread certain sections of the book. When I read a new book with a topic like this, I do read everything, but perhaps lightly skimming so that I can get through it and hold the whole picture in my head. Then I usually go back and read certain sections thoroughly, highlighting if I have a hard copy, taking notes if I am reading online. The point is I don't often get every single piece of information that the author has intended that I get. In case you skimmed certain parts, I am repeating some information or asking you to go back so that you get full use out of the worksheets.

Some of the examples I use to get you rolling with the worksheets may address weight loss goals as well as food plan goals. I personally started with keto only to get rid of my pre-diabetes. My main focus with my goals was how to stick to the food plan. As time went on and my A1c came out of the pre-diabetic range, I added weight loss goals when I was comfortable with eating keto and then low carb. Even though this is not a weight loss/diet book *per se*, I know many of you do have weight loss goals and so I want to include those discussions in the worksheets.

Some people find that it is *only* the food that drives them to eat. Once carbohydrates are reduced or eliminated and they eat more fat for satiety, the problem takes care of itself. I am not one of those people. My weight problem is as much between my ears as what insulin, ghrelin and leptin dictate. Therefore, although this is not a weight-loss book, but one designed to help you with keto or various stages of low carbohydrate eating using the *Granny Keto Transitions Program*™, I still want some of the worksheets and lessons to address head hunger issues like urges and self-talk. Also, please reread CHAPTER 4 (STEP 2, ELIMINATE GRAINS AND LEGUMES) for a discussion about bringing your family into the meal-planning process.

The worksheets here in PART 5 are called MEAL PLANNING AND SHOPPING, and they will help you with meal planning and grocery shopping.

Chapter Fifteen

Learning to Plan Keto Meals

I do not offer meal plans on my website or in my coaching. By that I mean actual meal plans that tell you what to eat for breakfast, lunch, dinner and snacks. I have always hated any diet that worked that way because I know what I like. If weighing and measuring is necessary, I can do that myself with a list of foods that I can choose from. I often say, "I don't let anyone tell me what to do, not even me." When I allow myself variety and free choice, I have a better chance of following a plan. I offer suggestions for how to make your own meal plans. In my opinion, specifics on when and what to eat are not a practical path to success. There are some actual meal-planning sites and if you feel most comfortable having someone tell you what and when to eat then a Google search will produce several.

I am going to give you the platform for keto meal planning and honestly, this will help you so much more because it helps you learn how to eat in any situation whether it be at a restaurant, a party or even if you open the fridge and there are very slim pickings. I am putting keto instructions for meal planning before presenting the low carb meal planning instructions in the following chapter, because while planning low carb meals, you build on the bones of keto meal planning.

To begin with, here are three levels of how to do keto with 20 grams of carbohydrates as your base. Use these keto-level examples for how to decide on planning your program.

Level 1: Strict Keto

Strict keto is 20 or less total or net grams of carbohydrates. That means you weigh, measure and track everything – even lettuce leaves. This might be the first stop on the train for you if you already have diabetes or are trying to help or reverse some other severe metabolic condition (like polycystic ovary syndrome). This is where I started, and it is the most diet-like of the three levels.

Level 2: Mix Total and Net Carbohydrates

The next level (Granny Keto's hybrid approach, explained earlier) is to mix total carbohydrates with the net carbohydrates from fresh, whole berries, vegetables and avocados to make a grand total of 20 grams of carbohydrates. Any carbohydrates other than from whole berries, vegetables or avocado are counted as total carbs. With berries, vegetables and avocados, take the net carbohydrate count and add it to total carbohydrate count, for a grand total of 20 grams. This sounds complicated (and diet-like), but it is very comfortable because you do not have to skimp as much on fresh produce as you would if you were at Level 1.

LEVEL 3: SKIP COUNTING SOME VEGETABLES

A third way to do keto is to not count leafy greens and other above-ground vegetables (as well as some of the below-ground low carb veggies like radishes). You can still set your limit to 20 total carbs (of all other food). Until I made a further transition into low carb eating, this is the way I followed keto for about two years. It is the least diet-like level for keto and gives you the most freedom while still having a sense of tracking in the back of your mind ("Does it look like this is enough protein?" "Do I have enough fat for the day?").

Pick which level of keto you would like to do. I worked my way through all three levels. I hope this shows you that there is no black or white and no perfect vs. all bad and that you do not have to be tied into one level or the other. Learn to dance and you will find what works best for you. More importantly, you will see that there is variation. I am not sure I would suggest changing up things on a daily basis unless you try one level and immediately hate it. But, if you are not totally happy with what you are doing, feel free to change your approach every few weeks to see what resonates best with you. I lost most of my weight on Level 1. If I wanted to give a push to the fastest weight loss, I would go back to that for a short period.

When I first started keto, I used Carb Manager. This is an app where you enter your food for macronutrient and calorie calculations, similar to other apps such as My Fitness Pal and Lose It. Even if you are aware of your carb intake and how your plate and day look like, this is a good way to get started at the beginning or to do spot checks if you are not losing the weight you would like. Carb Manager has a nice pie chart so you can see exactly what your plate looks like. Doing Level 2 with Carb Manager was pretty easy as you could see both total and net carbs. When I moved to Level 3 (skipping counting some vegetables), I just did not enter leafy greens at all. I found that I was pretty much balanced at each meal: About 7g carbs and 30 to 35g protein and the rest fat. CHAPTER 13, DANCING WITH LOW CARB AND KETO goes into detail about balancing your plate and balancing your meals to get the correct macronutrients for the day. This ability to look at your plate and know what your plate should look like is the steppingstone to no longer needing to weigh, measure and track your food.

If you have 50 or more pounds to lose, do not concern yourself with quantities right now, but work to learn hunger and fullness signals. There is nothing to be gained (except weight!) from loading your plate with six eggs scrambled in butter and a pound of bacon (yes, folks, people new to keto have done that) if you feel sick from being full. If you feel great and have energy the rest of the day – enjoy yourself but be very aware when such quantities become too much for you. Just because you can, doesn't mean you should.

My meal suggestions are given without specific quantities. Use your own best judgment. Base this judgment on how a certain *quantity* of a food makes you feel. For instance, I enjoy cream in my coffee, but a bowl of creamed soup will make me nauseous. Learn to pay attention to this for yourself.

Please go back to CHAPTER 10 to the Yes/No list of keto foods. Print it out. Circle or highlight what you like to eat. Again, as with my keto-level examples above, what follows is how I did my keto meal planning. Take the lessons and apply them to any eating plan you are following.

BREAKFAST

Starting with the list in CHAPTER 10, let's look at breakfast. My favorite breakfast is the night-before leftovers. Fish and broccoli might not float your boat at 7AM, so let's look at more common breakfast foods.

Eggs any which way are fine. If you are looking to add fat, go for eggs scrambled with cream and cooked in butter or ghee. On the side you can put bacon, salami, sausage, full-fat kielbasa, full-fat hot dogs, steak, etc. Whenever I scramble eggs, I always throw in a handful of baby spinach or sautéed mushrooms. If you are sensitive to chicken eggs, duck eggs may be a good substitution and are becoming more available in some markets. Very often people will have sensitivity to one but not the other. If you do eat eggs, make sure you search for the hundreds of keto crustless quiche recipes. These can be made into wonderful grab-and-go egg muffins with all sorts of goodness like ham, cheese, sausage, leeks and all sorts of other vegetables. Let's not forget hard-boiled eggs and egg salad!

After a certain point, especially if you were a cereal or baked-goods breakfast person, you may tire of eggs. Often, I have turkey breast rolled up in a cheese wrap, and countless mornings I have had ham and cheese rollups in lettuce leaves. One of my favorite breakfasts is a fried beef burger or chicken burger. There are several brands of keto granolas that do not contain wheat products and are made primarily of nuts and seeds, or you can make your own. Just be careful to count these as total carbs no matter what the fiber count is (unless you are counting net carbs only).

There are several full-fat plain yogurts and Greek yogurts that are very low in carbs. As mentioned earlier, it is okay to count only half of the carbohydrates present in plain full-fat yogurt. This is because yogurt products are labeled with their properties prior to the conversion of the milk to yogurt. Enzymes present in the process will convert the lactose to lactic acid. I pick a very low carb plain Greek yogurt and do not count it at all, as I have only a small amount – about ½ cup. To this I add seeds and nuts or keto granola, or cut-up cucumbers and mint (which, by the way, blended, makes a fabulous dressing). If you are eating berries, go ahead and add them to the yogurt, although I would save this combination – with a sprinkling of chopped nuts – for a wonderful dessert later in the day.

I have made stunning breakfast plates with smoked salmon, olives, one or two cheeses, radishes, celery sticks and sliced cucumber. A caprese salad is no more than sliced mozzarella, tomatoes, basil, balsamic vinaigrette and olive oil. Full-fat cottage cheese and ricotta cheese are allowed on keto, but make sure you count the carbs.

Even though I suggest not going with keto baked-good substitutes, you are highly unlikely to go overboard with these morning "coffee sides" that follow.

- Cloud bread: Google "cloud bread" or "oopsie rolls" and you will find dozens upon dozens of recipes and directions. Basically, it is just four ingredients: eggs, cream cheese, cream of tartar, and salt. I add cinnamon and a little sweetener for my morning recipe.

- Keto Egg Loaf with Blueberry and Lemon from the website Have Butter Will Travel, makes a wonderful breakfast. It is good enough for company. True story: I served it for a Thanksgiving brunch and as people were finishing it, I whipped up a second one. It was the hit of the brunch! It's great to grab-and-go or to enjoy leisurely at home.

- If I have a really strong hankering for a bagel there is a keto bagel recipe on my website at Miriamhatoum.com and you will find many more on the Internet. However, unlike the cloud bread and Keto Egg Loaf, there is a modicum of disappointment because although you can slather it with cream cheese and top it with tomatoes, onions and smoked salmon, it does not fool you into thinking you are eating a "real" bagel. However, if you miss bagels and really want to have something like that to hold in your hand, go for it!

- The new fave: CHAFFLES. Using a waffle maker, you can make these sweet or savory. There are hundreds of recipes on the Internet and there are Facebook pages devoted to them.

If you experiment with keto baked goods along your journey, you will develop less of a disconnect between your palate and your brain. You may actually enjoy the keto bagel.

The reason I call these few breakfast baked goods "unlikely to overeat baked coffee sides" in the worksheets that follow is because their sweetness factor is minimal, which often drives the "I can't stop eating this" behavior. Give me a keto cookie or cake or sweet Chaffles with Lakanto maple syrup, a monk fruit sweetener, and it's another story!

LUNCH

Lunch is what seems to stymie people new to keto. This is especially so if you work outside the home. The challenges you face might be that you need to pack lunch, often go out with colleagues or lunch is brought in. It poses a further problem if you are absolutely wedded to the idea that lunch is synonymous with sandwich.

Let me address sandwich solutions first because that might be the one thing that keeps you keto! I am not one to endorse products in this book, but right now as of the writing of this book, there is a product called Cheese Folio (and other brands are popping up) which is round and thin (like a tortilla) but is made from cheese. It is flexible, strong and can be filled with any of your preferred sandwich fillings. Cheese Folios pack well. On the Internet and in cookbooks you will find many recipes for keto "bread." Some of these hold up well to sandwich fillings and can be made into rolls as well as into sliceable breads. In the reference section at the end of this book I list some of my favorite cookbooks. Many of them have keto bread recipes. If you don't want to bake a bread, you can use lettuce leaves as your filling holder. I do suggest, however, that you pack your "holder" separately from the filling. Things tend to get soggy.

If you have a microwave at work or have a good wide-necked thermos, soups and stews make great lunches. Dinner leftovers are also wonderful, and *some* work well without reheating. I emphasize some because the high-fat content of a lot of the keto foods requires left-overs to be reheated. It's not necessary to reheat everything though. I am happy with a cold hamburger. Of course, you can have any of your breakfast items for lunch.

Take anything that you would use as a sandwich filling and just eat it cold without a wrap: tuna salad, egg salad, deli meat and cheese. There are plenty of canned foods that don't have to go into a sandwich. I never had a sardine until about two years into keto. OMG, where were they my entire life? Granted, it might not be something you like, but I have had many of my clients say, "Oh, I forgot about sardines." From there I went on to other canned fish, regular or smoked, including herring, trout and mackerel.

In PROTOCOL MEAL PLANNING (CHAPTER 17) you will see that my standard lunch, either while I was working or at home once I retired, was usually a salad every day. I did not enjoy this until I moved out of Level (1) of keto (counting all carbohydrates as total). My salads were still on the side-salad size in Level (2), but I thoroughly enjoyed meal-sized salads once I moved into Level (3) where not counting leafy greens became the way I ate. I did measure the carbohydrates for other salad ingredients, if I used them, such as tomatoes and carrots. I also tracked carbohydrates, protein and fats for dressings and proteins. What I did not count were the leafy greens and above-ground veggies like celery and cucumbers. I know I have promised you no weighing and measuring and freedom from diet prison but do this until you are familiar with using a particular food. Eventually weighing, measuring and tracking your food will become superfluous because of your knowledge and trust in your choices.

I rediscovered blue cheese dressing. It is so easy to make, but almost any quality brand will be fine if the carbohydrate count is about 1 to 2 carbs per two tablespoons. Some don't even have that many. I discovered ranch dressing for the first time. My favorite homemade dressing is two tablespoons of a good olive oil, one tablespoon of apple cider vinegar, about half teaspoon of Dijon mustard, a pinch of salt and a touch of sweetener.

To the salad I add any protein (usually left over from dinner the night before, like chicken or steak) and cheese if I want it. With my salads then (keto) and now (low carb) I make a mixture of equal parts: chopped walnuts, pumpkin seeds, sunflower seeds, half as much hemp hearts and chia seeds. I sprinkle on a couple of tablespoons of this, or, if I don't have any protein in the salad, I will put four tablespoons (a quarter cup). If you make your own mixture and want to carefully count carbohydrates at the beginning of your journey, weigh or measure each component and then divide the mixture as you want. Again, as with everything else, once you are aware of the carbohydrates you are consuming you will find you don't have to be as exact as you put a seed/nut concoction together. *Remember: Our goal is to get out of diet prison, not make the bars stronger!* Often, I will top the salad with just walnuts. Sometimes if a person is in a weight-loss stall, removing nuts and seeds is helpful to get the scale moving again but most often this is because they may not have tracked carefully when they first started the new food. Your handful is different from my handful. As a result, you may be eating more than you realize. Also, some people find that nuts and seeds may be inflammatory foods for them, which will also stall weight-loss efforts.

Having bouillon with butter at work was very helpful if I found I was hungry before my lunch hour or wanted to have something at the end of the day before my commute home. I would also have pickles, cut celery sticks and radishes at the ready. These all make good snacks. However, the longer I did keto and made higher-fat choices, I found that I was not hungry between meals.

What if your office is doing take-out? I always had something at work that I could go to like broth, canned fish, salami and cheese, and really, I was very rarely caught without my own lunch. If you choose the take-out, make your best choices. Steamed vegetables and chicken are always available from a Chinese restaurant. Taco filling with extra veggies and cheese without a shell is fine. Don't forget the guacamole and sour cream – both keto-approved foods. Pizza toppings scraped off the crust can work. Eat keto (or low carb) the rest of the day with either of these choices (taco or pizza) because there is usually more sugar in the tomato sauce and taco seasoning than there would be if you made the same foods at home. Deli sandwiches? PERFECT! Just ditch the roll and stay away from the potato salad. And ALWAYS remember: GOOD-BETTER-BEST (CHAPTERS 5, 12 and 20).

DINNER

If you go back to CHAPTER 13, DANCING WITH LOW CARB AND KETO, you can see there is a difference between working the steps and working the combinations. For learning to do keto dinners, start with the steps, as it is easiest on yourself and the family. If you love to cook and want to dive right in with recipes, go for it.

What do I mean by steps with regard to planning dinner? Take your elements in this order: protein, fat and carbohydrate. Decide on a protein choice: Meat, chicken or fish. Assess the fat content. If you are making short ribs, for instance, or having chicken thighs with skin, you might be all set for the fat that accompanies the protein. If you are eating something lean, make sure to enhance it with butter or cream sauce or prepare it in a nice avocado or olive oil. For instance, when I am making a skinless cut of chicken, I might put mayonnaise on it when I bake it or bake it in a cream sauce. Doing something like this is still working with steps, not necessarily recipes and combinations. Also looking at fats, feel free to fry things in bacon fat or butter, and enjoy some butter on steamed vegetables. For something green on the side, popular choices are string beans, Brussels sprouts or asparagus. Although it's not green, fried fresh cauliflower florets make a wonderful side dish. If I have not had salad at lunch, I usually serve one at dinner, but I take a side-salad portion, not a huge bowl like I would do if it was my main meal.

When looking at the carbohydrate portion of your meal, see what you have left in your carb count for the day and enjoy. When you make recipes there will be carb grams to factor in, but if you start with "steps" the food is plain enough and it will be easy to see if you have some left for the day. If you are counting carbohydrates at a Level (1) or Level (2) meal plan, remember that all vegetables and most dairy have carbohydrates. *If you are counting, then count.* Don't make the assumption that you won't go over your allowance just because it's a few extra string beans. If you have carbohydrate allowance left, you can use it on a dessert that might be berries or a keto treat. Some "treats" can be five or more carbs, so no matter what level you are following, be careful.

The carbohydrate portion of your dinner is where you can go to town if you are cooking for non-keto family and friends. Honestly, if you don't say anything to anyone, your friends and family might never know you are eating keto. Make your usual rice, pasta or potato. Serve fresh bread. Put some croutons on the table. Serve dessert. Keep your head about you and don't throw a pity party that you can't have this and that. With a determined attitude you are in no danger of eating all the other food once you make up your mind you are going to eat this way.

BREAKFAST WORKSHEET

- Eggs: Fried, poached, scrambled, hard-boiled, egg salad
- Omelets and Quiches made with
  - Cheese
  - Bacon
  - Salami
  - Kielbasa
  - Sausage
  - Hot dogs
  - Vegetables
- Rollups with any deli meat
- Sides of avocado and olives
- Keto or low-sugar granola
- Yogurt with
  - Keto Granola
  - Nuts and seeds
  - Cucumber and mint
  - Berries
- Caprese plate (mozzarella cheese, tomatoes, basil, olive oil and balsamic vinegar)
- Charcuterie plates with
  - Smoked salmon
  - Cheese
  - Meats such as salami and prosciutto
  - Olives
  - Vegetables
- Baked goods
  - Keto Selections
  - Other:
  - Other:

What are some of your own ideas?

- Ways to make eggs
- Sides and mix-ins for eggs
- Rollup ideas
- Yogurt mix-in ideas
- Combination Plates

LUNCH WORKSHEET

- "Holders"
  - Keto Breads and rolls
  - Cheese Wraps
  - Soft-leaf lettuce for rollups

- Fillings
  - Tuna salad
  - Egg salad
  - Deli meat
  - Cheese
  - Other:
  - Other:

- Other proteins (that don't require heating)
  - Canned fish like sardines, trout, herring, mackerel
  - Hard-boiled eggs
  - Sliced chicken, sliced steak, left-over fish
  - Other:
  - Other:

- Salad toppings
  - Any of the above
  - Nuts and seeds
  - Other:

- Dressings
  - Olive oil/vinegar
  - Other:
  - Other:

- If heating or thermos is available
  - Soups
  - Stews
  - Any leftovers that are best hot or warm

- Snacks
  - Bouillon (with butter)
  - Celery sticks and radishes
  - Pickles
  - Salami and cheese
  - Salsa or guacamole with cheese "wisps"
  - Olives
  - Other:
  - Other:

Your Favorites:

DINNER WORKSHEET

What follows below will help you understand what I mean by "working the steps" vs. "working the combinations." In addition, these two processes will help you sort through some of the confusion about what to make, especially if you are planning meals for other people.

WORKING THE STEPS TO MAKE DINNER		
(In this section list the proteins and fats that you like to eat)		
PROTEIN	**FATS**	**CARBOHYDRATES**
		(In this section put keto carbs (K) and also non-keto (NK) carbs that the family would like)
Roast chicken	Butter for veggies, dressing	K: cauliflower; NK: rice pilaf
Grilled hamburgers	Mayonnaise, blue cheese	K: onions, tomatoes, and pickles; NK: buns
Boiled lobster	Lots of butter!	K: salad; NK: baked potato

RECIPES (COMBINATIONS) THAT YOU AND THE FAMILY WOULD LIKE

Here are some of my family favorites. There are thousands of recipes on the Internet, hundreds of keto cookbooks (my favorites are in the reference section) and don't forget – without anyone's help you can probably make changes yourself to make your favorite recipes keto-compliant.

RECIPES	CAN I MAKE THIS KETO?	WHERE CAN I FIND A RECIPE IF I NEED IT?
Fried chicken (baked)	Yes	miriamhatoum.com
Tacos	Yes	*A Journey Worth Taking*. Kristie Sullivan
Mac'n cheese	Yes	stellastyle.com
Crustless quiche	Yes	I can figure it out!

Build on these lists. Honestly, you, your family and friends won't be missing anything if you make a good-faith effort to keep an open mind and try new things. There is even keto low-sugar wine and entire cookbooks devoted to things like keto cocktails and keto ice cream.

Chapter Sixteen

Learning to Plan Low Carb Meals

This chapter is almost identical to the previous chapter, Learning to Plan Keto Meals. Build on the "bones" of keto. There are some slight changes but for the most part, the information you learned in the previous chapter on Learning to Plan Keto Meals, holds as well for Learning to Plan Low Carb Meals.

When planning your low carb meals, allow for variety in how you approach it. For instance, on Step 1 of Transitions, you may be allowing packaged goods where sugar might be very low on the ingredient list or you may be eating only naturally occurring sugars (like fruit) and not adding any type of sugar to your foods. On Step 2 of Transitions, if are you looking to eat only gluten-free, it means you may allow some of the grains. On Step 3 of Transitions, you may be heading towards keto and prefer to not use your carbohydrate allowance for things like bread. If you are on Step 3 but *not* heading to keto you may be eating all foods but making sure you are within a reasonable carbohydrate range. Each step of the *Granny Keto Transitions Program*™ can incorporate different levels just as with the keto levels in the previous chapter.

Similar Strategies to Keto Meal Planning

- Similar to levels of keto, decide how many grams of carbohydrates you would like to have in a day.
- Decide whether you are leaving out any specific foods. Are you following one of *Granny Keto Transitions Program*™ Steps, and what variations might you have within those?
- List the foods that you and your family like the best.
- List your favorite recipes and see if they need to be tweaked to fit your food plan.
- Separate out (for now) breakfast, lunch, dinner and snack ideas.

Different Strategies

- When you are planning your family meals, unless you are leaving out certain foods (i.e., sugars, grains, legumes, starchy vegetables, etc.), you can pretty much plan your meals to include everything. However, if you do that, it becomes more important to watch portion sizes than when doing keto. Although you should still eat to your hunger scale, be aware that certain carbohydrate-containing foods do not fill you up the way protein and fat would. For instance, if you want something like pasta, it is best to portion it out and count the carbohydrates before you start eating. This is especially important if you are skipping directly to Step 3 (eating low carb), and your only concern is carbohydrate grams, not the specific foods.

- When you are planning your snacks, it is important to pick filling food choices that include protein and fat, otherwise, you might be hungry almost immediately. A candy bar or popcorn might be nice treats if you can fit them in to your carbohydrate allowance, but they raise insulin, and you will get hungry sooner. When you are planning snacks for the week, try not to include high starch or sugary items more than once or twice.

The following meal worksheets are based on the bones of keto. You will add choices based on which *Granny Keto Transitions Program*™ step you are on, as well as personal choices and preferences. You will also make your choices as to whole foods vs. packaged and prepared foods. I encourage whole, natural foods when available. If you are not eating keto, pay attention to the amount of fat and salt you eat. They don't mix well health-wise with carbohydrate.

As you fill out the worksheets on the next few pages here is some more guidance for eating low carb in way that will truly and permanently free you from diet prison. As stated at the beginning of this chapter, build on the bones of keto. That means take the keto principles that were presented in *Granny Keto Transitions Program*™.

- First, think in terms of elimination. No sugar, baked goods, grains, legumes, fruit (except berries) or starchy vegetables. Make sure you eat adequate protein and fat so you will not be hungry between meals. These are the bones.

- Add to the bones some non-keto foods of your choice.

- No more than once per meal, and preferably no more than twice per day, add to your meal something that is limited because of the carbohydrate count such as rice, pasta, bread, starchy vegetables or legumes. If you want that sandwich at lunch, enjoy, but consider it two carb choices (each piece of bread being one) and have only one more carb choice at another meal.

- Once or twice a week, if you want, have something with sugar such as a baked good or something else that is sweet. This can be for a dessert or a special occasion (like a piece of birthday cake). Watch your portion size! Take half of what you would have taken in the olden days.

- Keep your fruit selections to no more than two a day, and preferably not dried fruit or tropical fresh fruit. When you do choose dried fruit or tropical fresh fruit have only one fruit selection that day.

BREAKFAST WORKSHEET

- Eggs: Fried, poached, scrambled, hard-boiled, egg salad
- Omelets and Quiches made with
  - Cheese
  - Bacon
  - Salami
  - Kielbasa
  - Sausage
  - Hot dogs
  - Vegetables
- Rollups with any deli meat
- Sides of avocado and olives
- Keto or low-sugar granola
- Yogurt with
  - Keto Granola
  - Nuts and seeds
  - Cucumber and mint
  - Berries
- Caprese plate (mozzarella cheese, tomatoes, basil, olive oil and balsamic vinegar)
- Charcuterie plates with
  - Smoked salmon
  - Cheese
  - Meats such as salami and prosciutto
  - Olives
  - Vegetables
- Baked goods
  - Keto Selections
  - Other:
  - Other:

What are some of your own ideas?

- Ways to make eggs
- Sides and mix-ins for eggs
- Rollup ideas
- Yogurt mix-in ideas
- Combination Plates

LUNCH WORKSHEET

- "Holders"
  - Keto Breads and rolls
  - Cheese Wraps
  - Soft-leaf lettuce for rollups

- Fillings
  - Tuna salad
  - Egg salad
  - Deli meat
  - Cheese
  - Other:
  - Other:

- Other proteins (that don't require heating)
  - Canned fish like sardines, trout, herring, mackerel
  - Hard-boiled eggs
  - Sliced chicken, sliced steak, left-over fish
  - Other:
  - Other:

- Salad toppings
  - Any of the above
  - Nuts and seeds
  - Other:

- Dressings
  - Olive oil/vinegar
  - Other:
  - Other:

- If heating or thermos is available
  - Soups
  - Stews
  - Any leftovers that are best hot or warm

- Snacks
  - Bouillon (with butter)
  - Celery sticks and radishes
  - Pickles
  - Salami and cheese
  - Salsa or guacamole with cheese "wisps"
  - Olives
  - Other:
  - Other:

DINNER WORKSHEET

(See example Dinner Worksheet in the previous chapter.)

WORKING THE STEPS TO MAKE DINNER		
PROTEIN	**FATS**	**CARBOHYDRATES** In this section put keto carbs (K) and also non-keto (NK) carbs that the family would like

RECIPES (COMBINATIONS) THAT YOU AND THE FAMILY WOULD LIKE

RECIPES	CAN I MAKE THIS KETO?	WHERE CAN I FIND A RECIPE IF I NEED IT?

Build on these lists. Honestly, you, your family and friends won't be missing anything if you make a good-faith effort to keep an open mind and try new things.

Chapter Seventeen

Protocol Meal Planning

Your True Escape From Diet Prison

Protocol or template meal planning is my most favorite way of meal planning. It uses Granny Keto's Dancing and Kissing methods (Chapters 13 and 14, respectively). It ultimately requires no weighing, measuring or tracking. It does, however, assume that if you are new to carb counting, that you do weigh, measure and track your favorite keto foods until you learn the protein, fat and carbohydrate gram counts for them. This also works perfectly for low carb eating. You will eventually learn when enough is enough of each macronutrient. I always check new foods and make no assumptions. If you are doing Steps 1 and 2 of *Granny Keto Transitions Program*™, you need only eat to your hunger scale, eliminating any foods you are cutting out at each step. If you are at the beginning of Step 3 (low carb) you may want to weigh, measure and track your carbohydrates. For instance, at the beginning when I had a salad, I also listed the types of greens and other vegetables, the dressing, nuts, feta cheese and olives. Eventually it just became MY SALAD. As you use protocol meal planning more and more, it will become easier and easier to make choices based on your new knowledge and it will also become second nature to trust yourself. You will be off that dang roller coaster and out of diet prison forever. I promise! And, my friend, you will not even have to do the protocol planning once you get the hang of things.

At the beginning, I did protocol meal planning for the week so that I could look it over to make sure I was eating enough chicken and fish, with red meat and lamb a few times during the week. For keto, I could also look at a meal and realize that it would need butter or a cream sauce or a side vegetable. I was also able to keep track of whether I was eating the same thing all the time. Sometimes I would make a note that I needed to try a new recipe or two. I found it different from regular meal planning because by the time I got the hang of it, it was just an outline and that is all I needed. I was dancing with keto and could size up a meal choice and know if it would fit perfectly into my day or even my week.

Protocol Meal Planning Worksheet

Early protocol planning: My early protocol planning was like regular meal planning, but it allowed me to move toward what you see in the second example. In my earlier keto protocols (you can also use this method for low carb meal plans) I included the protein, fat and carbohydrate count.

Eventually (as you will see from the next example), I counted only carbohydrates if a food was an add-on like the nuts or salad dressing, a snack item like cheese wisps or a recipe where the carbs are accounted for. I did this on Level 3 of keto eating and planning (CHAPTER 15), where I already no longer counted leafy green and above-ground vegetables. The following macro counts are for the brands that I used (sometimes food will have a "generic" count, but a lot times the carbohydrate count varies by brand).

Breakfast: 2 mugs of coffee with 2 TBS heavy cream each; 2 eggs scrambled in 1 TBS butter; Chopped mushrooms, leeks and peppers, baby spinach; 4 strips of bacon

Protein: 26.4   Fat: 57.4   Carbohydrates: 2.9

Lunch: Salad with 2 TBS chopped walnuts, 6 olives, 1 oz. feta cheese, 4 cherry tomatoes, 2 TBS Ranch dressing, 2 oz cubed salami

Protein: 12.9   Fat: 51.9   Carbohydrates: 12.3 (Each cherry tomato has 1 carb)

Dinner: Granny Keto's "fried" chicken, small salad with 1 TBS blue cheese dressing; string beans with 1 TBS butter

Protein: 48   Fat: 40.5   Carbohydrates: <1

Snack 1: Mug of broth with 1 TBS butter; 10 cheese wisps

Protein: 7   Fat: 7   Carbohydrates: <1

Snack 2: ½ cup of plain Greek yogurt with ½ cup mixed berries

Protein: 12.7   Fat: 3   Carbohydrates: 9

I put this day here so that you could see where it needs some tweaking. This might be a little heavy on the protein for you (107 grams), but it is great for the fat (159.8) and almost right on the money for the carbs (24.2, *total* carbs not counting the greens; if I left off the tomatoes it would have been **20 total** carbs). When you are starting with keto, you do not have to worry about protein – just keep your carbs low. If you are going to start counting protein, then for a day like this I do not suggest cutting back on the chicken because in quantity it was not a lot (just 2 pieces). What I would tweak is perhaps cutting the yogurt out and only having berries, and maybe having two slices of bacon instead of four. Or I would keep the plan just as is, but the next day pick a dinner that is a little lighter on protein so that every few days it evens out. As much as we want to adhere to the basic "rules" of keto to get the best results, we are not machines and can vary a little bit day to day as long as things even out for the week. I will repeat something here that is very important. If you have diabetes, non-alcoholic fatty liver disease, insulin resistance, polycystic ovary syndrome or any other metabolic disorder that would benefit from eating keto, then you might want to follow counts even more closely than I am suggesting here. Also let me add, that as you do keto longer, you will be less hungry and eat less, so counts will take care of themselves without a lot of worry and tweaking.

More experienced protocol planning was just sticking to a Yes/No list (CHAPTER 10) and eventually I did not even add the carbohydrate gram count. I knew from several days, if not weeks, of the early protocol planning, approximately what my other macros would be. I just needed to double-check to make sure my carbs were low.

BREAKFAST: Coffee, scrambled eggs with vegetables and bacon. (Carbs: 2.9)

LUNCH: MY salad. (Carbs: 12.3 – remember tomatoes are carb-heavy; you can leave them out and just have greens.)

DINNER: Granny Keto's fried chicken with side vegetable and butter. (Carbs: <1)

SNACK 1:   Mug of broth with butter; 10 cheese wisps. (Carbs: <1)

SNACK 2:   Plain Greek yogurt with berries. (Carbs: 9)

Most experienced protocol planning might be just the awareness that you are eating a keto (or low carb) meal with your hunger scale at a 4 to 6. ***You are now dancing! THIS is the TRUE lifestyle. You are no longer in diet prison!***

To begin this process for yourself it is best to treat it like "real" meal planning and count protein, fat and carbohydrates until you really have a handle on, and knowledge of, what you are eating in a day. Just because a food is on the Yes/No list doesn't mean it does not have carbs. Especially if you are starting out at Level (1) or Level (2) with total carb or net carb count, it is very important that you know where those carbs come from. Dairy has carbs. Lettuce has carbs. Zucchini and string beans have carbs. If you decide to move to Level (3) you can relax on counting every leafy green or above-ground vegetable carb, but remember others can creep in. In keto lingo it is called "Carb Creep." It is very real!

PROTOCOL MEAL PLANNING WORKSHEETS

Breakfast:

PROTEIN:____FAT:____CARBOHYDRATES:____

Lunch:

PROTEIN:____FAT:____CARBOHYDRATES:____

Dinner:

PROTEIN:____FAT:____CARBOHYDRATES:____

Snack 1:

PROTEIN:____FAT:____CARBOHYDRATES:____

Snack 2:

PROTEIN:____FAT:____CARBOHYDRATES:____

_____

Breakfast:

PROTEIN:____FAT:____CARBOHYDRATES:____

Lunch:

PROTEIN:____FAT:____CARBOHYDRATES:____

Dinner:

PROTEIN:____FAT:____CARBOHYDRATES:____

Snack 1:

PROTEIN:____FAT:____CARBOHYDRATES:____

Snack 2:

PROTEIN:____FAT:____CARBOHYDRATES:____

_____

Breakfast:

PROTEIN:____FAT:____CARBOHYDRATES:____

Lunch:

PROTEIN:____FAT:____CARBOHYDRATES:____

Dinner:

PROTEIN:____FAT:____CARBOHYDRATES:____

Snack 1:

PROTEIN:____FAT:____CARBOHYDRATES:____

Snack 2:

PROTEIN:____FAT:____CARBOHYDRATES:____

CHAPTER EIGHTEEN

GROCERY SHOPPING

When people first start grocery shopping for keto or any new way of eating, they tend to find it expensive. It can be, but it does not need to be. These are things that can make it expensive:

- You buy grass-fed and pasture-raised meat (not necessary).
- You buy only pasture-raised eggs (not necessary).
- You buy only organic vegetables and berries (not necessary).
- You hunt down carb-free (sugar free/nitrate free) processed meats (not necessary).
- You are still buying a lot of junk food for the rest of the family.
- You buy too much food.
- You buy all the cookbooks and start ordering strange and unusual ingredients from Amazon.

Although it is wonderful if your food budget allows grass-fed, pasture-raised and organic meats and produce, you do not have to have these things to be successful on keto (or any step of *Granny Keto Transitions Program*™). Regular produce, meats and eggs are fine. When you start to save a lot of money on your grocery bills you can roll over the savings into better-quality foods or you can go on a trip to Hawaii wearing that new bathing suit you will soon fit into! You do not need top-shelf expensive food.

Regarding the second half of the list, if you are buying more meats, cheeses and produce for yourself and loading up on junk food your bill might be a little higher. The problem is not keto or low carb. The problem is what you are buying for your family. How about less pre-frozen meals, cereals and other standard breakfast foods? How about fewer snacks and instead prepare hardier meals so the kids won't be looking to eat all the time? We stopped going to bakeries for pastries and fresh bread. I stopped the take-out coffees with bagels and muffins. I brought lunch to work instead of take-out and fast food. I planned for dinners (and meal prepped quite a bit on the weekends) so I would have something ready when I got home from a long day at work. Your intention to have Bolognaise sauce with zoodles is not going to happen if you have to start chopping vegetables and cooking after an eight-hour day at work and a one-hour commute, with or without kids waiting for you when you walk through the door. All these savings can be rolled back into your grocery budget.

You will also find that as you are really into the swing of eating the ketogenic way, or even one of the TRANSITIONS steps, you will not be as hungry and will automatically buy less food. I threw out a lot of fresh food: vegetables, berries, fish and even salami and cheese which you would think do not spoil, but they do. I learned that I very rarely wanted breakfast and that coffee would do. I maybe would have a piece of salami with a pickle mid-day at work or before leaving to go home, but very rarely wanted anything else that I brought with me. I did often make broth with a little bit of butter and put it into a to-go cup to enjoy all the way home. It was perfect! If you remember what I wrote earlier: My husband and I would buy two one-pound steaks for dinner. Eventually we shared the one. Further along the way, we would share the one steak, but I would still have some left over from my half and that is what I would cut up to put on my salad the next day. Our grocery bill started to go down with no effort.

The last thing I want to address are all the cookbooks and all the recipes. I bought so many keto baking ingredients I ended up giving them all away. I even paid for postage to mail things to friends in other parts of the country who were doing keto. That being said, three years later I repurchased some of these things because I was finally ready to branch out into baked goods. Not that you won't be ready at the very start of your keto journey if baking floats your boat, but this was an unwise direction for me. Also trying every new complicated recipe might not be your best way to start out. What follows is my own experience with keto and low carb baked goods and sweets, and also my take on starting with complicated recipes.

First of all, I hadn't learned yet: *Whatever you do, never run back to what broke you.* When I first started keto, I was excited about the keto breads, keto cookies, keto cakes, keto candy and keto ice cream (God help me…I bought an ice cream maker!). I was thinking that as long as something was keto, I could eat it. After all, the experts said that it was food itself that causes you to overeat. At some level this is true. When you eat foods that trigger your insulin your ghrelin (hunger hormone) goes up and your leptin (fullness hormone) goes down. If you eat keto, and your hormones start to regulate, you will not be hungry. This is true. However, what I neglected to understand is that I have a two-pronged problem. Yes, I had high fasting insulin and I was insulin resistant. That means that if I ate a slice of bread, my *body* craved the whole loaf. If I ate a cookie, my *body* craved the whole bag. I thought my forever happy ending would be to eat keto and never crave or overeat certain foods again. What I didn't realize that no amount of keto eating would solve my head hunger and "concept cravings." What I mean by "concept cravings" is that I wanted the cookies because they were cookies. The fact that they were high in fat and contained no wheat had no effect on my head hunger. I had a friend who suffered only from physical hunger. She could eat one sweetened fat bomb and not want to eat for hours. I saw it as candy and was driven to eat the entire batch. If this issue resonates with you, this is one reason I would tell you to stay away from all the recipes and cookbooks until you have your physical hunger under control and you do some of the thought work (coming up in the next part of this book).

Another reason I would recommend staying away from all the recipes and cookbooks when you are starting out on keto (or low carb) is so you can learn how various foods feel in your body.

It is important to learn how the elements of a recipe work for you. For instance, a high-fat recipe might not sit comfortably with you. Or some people never know they have dairy or egg or nut sensitivities until they start eating keto. Eating foods in their less complex state can give you a chance to really tune into what makes you not feel well as opposed to what makes your body hum and fill you with energy.

A third reason I would suggest you stay away from complex recipes at the start is my deep belief in my dancing and kissing approaches to learning this way of eating (CHAPTERS 13 AND 14, respectively) or any of the *Granny Keto Transitions Program*™ steps way of eating. What I truly want for you is to learn to live your life without weighing, measuring and tracking. The simpler you keep things at the beginning, the faster your trajectory will be to reaching your goals.

Dispelling the myths about what you must buy (organic, pasture-raised and grass-fed), cutting back on take-out, fast food and junk snacks, learning how much food you really need to eat and *slowly* building your pantry with unusual items for cooking and baking, will all go a long way to stretch your food budget and make shopping for keto no more expensive, and actually less expensive, than shopping for any other way of eating.

If you go back to CHAPTER 11 (QUESTIONS AND DISPELLING MYTHS) you will find more information to assure you that grocery shopping for keto (or low carb) does not have to be expensive and difficult. Also, if you learn to make your grocery list for the week, you can cut out a lot of extra purchases that will add up to quite a bit of money. Disciplined list-making and grocery shopping will pay off, not only in your pocket, but in the amount of confusion that may arise when starting a new eating plan. If you have never planned your grocery shopping the way I outline below, it might take a while to get used to, but I promise you, it will pay off in both saving time and money.

GROCERY SHOPPING WORKSHEET

Print out your meal plan worksheets. Have a blank sheet of paper. Every time a food is on one of the meal plans put the ingredients for it on the blank sheet of paper. Then arrange it according to food types and add quantities.

When I shop for the whole week, my first pass-through looks at all the meals and recipes I will be making and I just jot down what I need: one onion for this, two onions for that, one onion I will need during the week for my salad, and so the final list will have four onions. That way I rarely have to go out for anything other than my one grocery trip a week. I do have the time to go to the store every day, but I have found it better to concentrate on shopping for the week all at one time even if it means going to several different markets on the same day. If you do not already do a once-a-week grocery haul, then break it up into 2 or 3 trips – but don't go every day. Once a week is actually very efficient and saves money. I will use my early protocol meal plan above. The preliminary grocery list would be:

Eggs	Cream	Butter	Bacon
Mushrooms	Onions	Bell pepper	Baby spinach
Chopped walnuts	Black olives	Feta cheese	Cherry tomatoes
Mesclun mix	Romaine lettuce	Ranch dressing	Unsliced salami
Chicken legs	BBQ baked pork rinds	Avocado oil	Olive oil
SB bouillon	Cheese wisps	Pickles	Greek yogurt
Blueberries	Strawberries	Blackberries	Radishes
Celery	Cucumbers	Leeks	String beans

This list takes care of my breakfasts and lunches for the week if I am basically taking the same thing every day. I might vary my salads or change up the way I am making my eggs. I included the ingredients for one dinner recipe ("fried" chicken). However, your grocery list would be for the entire week. You would list what you need for everything, including snacks for other days and variations on your breakfasts and lunches.

The second, and maybe final, list would look like this, including, for this example, just the one dinner.

DAIRY	PRODUCE	MEATS	OTHER
1 dozen eggs	Mushrooms	2 packages bacon	Black olives
1 quart heavy cream	Onions	Chicken legs and thighs (8 pieces total)	Ranch dressing
1 pound butter	Leeks	Salami	Olive oil
Feta cheese	Bell peppers		Avocado oil
Greek yogurt	Romaine lettuce		Pickles
	Mesclun mix		Seitenbacher® (SB) vegetable bouillon
	Radishes		Cheese wisps
	Cucumbers		Chopped walnuts
	Celery		
	Cherry tomatoes		
	String beans		
	Strawberries		
	Blueberries		
	Blackberries		
	(add quantities to your liking)		

Now practice writing down EVERYTHING you need for your meals. For now, assume there won't be much variance in breakfasts and lunches. Include ingredients for at least one dinner. This is just practice for now.

Now put the items into categories with quantities.

DAIRY	PRODUCE	MEATS	OTHER

Here is a blank grocery-planning list. If you cannot look that far ahead into a full week, try three days. Part of the reason people don't like to grocery shop is because they are not organized. This should help! Not that I am bragging, but I can be done with a week's shopping in probably 20 to 30 minutes with this system.

List items needed after surveying your fridge and cabinets for staples you might need in addition to shopping for your meal plan. Also, take the list and check what you might have in your cabinets or fridge and cross out what you don't need. This prevents double-buying or having to go out a second time.

Arrange for category and quantity. I added household because I want you to plan a real list!

DAIRY	PRODUCE	MEATS	OTHER	HOUSEHOLD

Practice again but this time for 3 to 7 days. List items for your Protocol or Full Meal Plans including family items:

Arrange for category and quantity.

DAIRY	PRODUCE	MEATS	OTHER	HOUSEHOLD

PART SIX
NEW HABITS AND THOUGHTS

- Your Why
- Goal Setting
- Kaisen
- Circumstance-Thoughts-Feelings-Actions-Results (CTFAR)
- Recognizing and Sitting with Urges
- Self-Talk
- Mindfulness Practices
- Your Relationship with Yourself

The group of worksheets in this part is called NEW HABITS AND THOUGHTS. These are important items in your toolbox to help you set your WHY, and your goals. This toolbox will show you how to make improvements as you go along. The worksheets will help you work through thought patterns and processes which lead you to eat when you are not actually hungry, concepts often referred to as head hunger and heart hunger. Read through these even if you find that changing your food choices is all it takes for you to erase years of SAD (Standard American Diet) eating, as these are concepts that will help you be successful with any new way of eating and any life lesson. Have fun!

CHAPTER NINETEEN

YOUR WHY

Finding your WHY, the reason you are motivated and determined to find a new way of eating, is the touchstone for a successful transition to a new lifestyle. Your WHY can be ever-changing. There are many valid WHYs. You are entitled to as many or as few as you want. You can have more than one WHY and your WHY can change whether or not you have seen your first WHY to its conclusion. You will see in the process below that sometimes finding your WHY can follow many steps. Any one of those steps alone can be a fine WHY. You just have to dig until you make sure you are on board with the right WHY for you at the time.

Your WHY is very much like goal setting (in the next chapter). You can be vague to a point, but sometimes you will be better served if you are very specific. Also, as you narrow down the specificity of the WHY you sometimes get to the rock bottom of what will keep you on track. Let's follow this process to get to the ultimate WHY – but it is entirely possible that each WHY can stand alone. Explore the process so that you can see that there might be more behind a WHY than you think!

- I want to lose weight.
- I want to lose weight so I will look good in clothes.
- I want to look good in clothes so I will like what I see in the mirror.
- I want to like what I see in the mirror because then I will feel better about myself.
- I want to feel better about myself because then I will like myself.
- I want to like myself so that I can do better for myself.
- I want to do better for myself so that I can be proud that I honor my commitments to myself.
- I want to honor my commitments to myself because that is the kind of person I want to be.

The ultimate WHY in this example is "I want to be the kind of person who feels good about herself and who honors her commitments and sees things through." However, sometimes a WHY needs no process such as in my initial WHY: "I want to follow this program because I need to lower my blood sugar to a healthy range."

- When I started keto, my only WHY was to bring down my fasting blood sugar, which I did, and remarkably so.

- Then I wanted to learn all I could about keto and live the lifestyle to become a coach which was my next WHY, and I did it.

- My next WHY was to incorporate my years of being a dance instructor into my coaching program, which I did when I wrote Dancing with Low Carb and Keto.

- Then my WHY became that I wanted to see it through and stop weighing, measuring and tracking, which I did by coming up with my Protocol Meal Planning.

Each of these had goals attached to them, but I had to have the WHYs in the first place in order to formulate my goals. Many times during this journey I lost my way, but mostly because I lost my WHY. I had the piece of bread or the dessert because I had forgotten that keeping my blood sugar low was an important WHY. Or I got careless with my Protocol Meal Planning because I forgot the earlier WHY of wanting to be a good coach who lives the lifestyle she teaches.

In this example, the goal was to do Protocol Meal Planning every day. The WHY was because I wanted to live the keto lifestyle to be a good coach.

I have mentioned elsewhere that we are not machines, and sometimes living in the Land of Good Enough is about as perfect as it is going to get. This does not mean that you should not strive for better and best. It just means that as you pass through good enough that you don't need to beat yourself up for being there. And also, the expression "Life Happens" does mean that life happens, and try as we might, we get sidetracked. However, the stronger our WHYs and the more we keep them in front of our face and forefront in our mind, the less chance of being sidetracked no matter what happens.

On the WHY worksheet (Part 1), write out all the WHYs you can think of and whether or not they need a process. Then on the WHY worksheet (Part 2), go back and number them according to priority and importance to you. Get some index cards and write either one WHY on several cards or use several cards to list several WHYs. Put them in your kitchen, your office, your bedroom, the car and anywhere else you will look at them.

THEN, LOOK AT THEM! DAILY. MEAL BY MEAL if that will help you. Revise them and shuffle them around. Add new ones. And while you are at it, take some of the "positive replacements" from your Self-Talk worksheet in CHAPTER 24, and put those on index cards as well. Read these out loud. Punch a hole into the corner of each card and take the packs you have made for each room and run a ribbon through them. Read them like a book. Read them to your infant as a bedtime story. Make this project a living and breathing part of who you are and who you are going to become. When you tell yourself that you are someone who keeps commitments, you will become someone who keeps commitments.

There is a concept called cognitive dissonance. This means that there is a disconnect between what you believe you are, and how you really are. People innately strive to avoid inconsistent and conflicting beliefs with regard to their behavior. I always told my dancers: If you come out on stage with your head held high, a smile on your face and act as if you own the stage, you will someday own the stage.

You can either believe it when you see it, or you can see it when you believe it. Daily reading of your WHYs and of your positive self-talk will have you behaving as if they are already true. Believe in your results first, and you will see the results you want.

WHY WORKSHEET (Part 1)

In the first part of this space, write your WHYs – all of them. Don't worry right now about prioritizing them. Give some thought to whether they would be better served by going through the process such as the one at the beginning of this chapter. The list of WHYs at the beginning of this chapter can also all be single WHYs and not necessarily a process.

WHY:

      Process?

WHY:

      Process?

WHY:

      Process?

WHY:

      Process?

WHY:

      Process?

WHY:

      Process?

WHY WORKSHEET (Part 2)

Now take those WHYs from Part 1 and list them here:

WHY:

WHY:

WHY:

WHY:

WHY:

Number them according to priority and relist them now in order:

WHY:

WHY:

WHY:

WHY:

WHY:

With each one put at least one positive self-talk comment (example: WHY: I want to bring down my blood sugar. STATEMENT: I am worth it, and I can do it this time). Now go put them on index cards!

WHY:

     Affirmation:

WHY:

     Affirmation:

WHY:

     Affirmation:

WHY:

     Affirmation:

WHY:

     Affirmation:

Chapter Twenty

Goal Setting

Goal Setting is different from your WHY. Establishing your WHYS helps you with the overall reason for a lifestyle change, but it will take setting goals to know that you are making the transition successfully. When we lived in Brooklyn, New York, I remember going to Madison Square Garden to see wrestling. Wrestlers were usually on our television a half dozen times a week and I knew them all. In the 1990s there was an up-and-coming wrestler, Diamond Dallas Page. He is the founder of a wonderful program called DDPY (Diamond Dallas Page Yoga) that started as "Yoga for Regular Guys" or "Not Your Mama's Yoga." He has a great goal-setting technique that he refers to as SMACK DOWN (which is a wrestling reference). Here it is:

Make your goals:

S   Specific

M   Measurable

A   Achievable

C   Compatible

K   Keep it going

      D   Do it

      O   Own it

      W   Write it down

      N   **NOW**

Using my interpretations of how to use SMACK DOWN, let's explore each of these elements.

SPECIFIC: The way to work on a goal is to make it very specific. You might say: "My goal is to lose weight" or "My goal is to look good in clothes." Both are admirable goals but will get you nowhere. Be specific: "My goal is to lose 50 pounds" or "My goal is to fit into my blue dress for the wedding."

MEASURABLE: Decide on the number of pounds to lose or the dress size you want to buy. It can also be something else unrelated to weight loss, such as how many steps you want to take or how many hours you want to aim to sleep each night. In this example, however, I am going to work with weight loss and dress size. Have the goal be measurable: "I have looked at the calendar and I know that at a healthy rate of two pounds a week, it is conceivable that I can lose 24 pounds in the three months for the wedding I am going to." "If I lose 20 to 24 pounds, or even 15 pounds, in three months, I know I can fit into my size 16 dress for the wedding."

ACHIEVABLE: Look at the calendar and then look at your lifestyle. See what can fit and what cannot fit. Fifty pounds in three months might be achievable if you barely eat and exercise all day, but is that likely to happen with the way you live your life? NO! Achievable: Would 15 to 24 pounds be achievable if you (1) cut out snacks and night-time eating, (2) drink water instead of all that coffee and soda and (3) go walking on your lunch hour to make that goal achievable? YES! If you lost those 15 pounds, would fitting into a dress smaller by one to two sizes be achievable? YES!

COMPATIBLE: As in the example above, look at the compatibility of your life with your goals. You may find it easy enough to cut out the snacking, drink more water and walk at lunch with the way you live your day, even with getting kids off to school in the morning, going to work, then coming home to homework, dinner and bedtime routines. Compatible? YES! Now let's look at that dress for another layer of compatibility. You have a dress that you love in your closet that is two sizes too small. Is it achievable that you drop those two dress sizes in three months? Yes… BUT: you bought this dress five years ago before you had and breastfed two children and although you can go into a store and buy that size, is your bustline still compatible with those buttons? Okay, we can laugh, but compatibility takes on many forms and you need to be open to the fact that sometimes a goal is just not compatible in some way, shape or form.

KEEP IT GOING: Pick a goal that you can sustain. If you have made your goal achievable and compatible, chances are you can see it through, but life happens and sometimes you can't get out for those walks or cook dinner. For now, leave the Land of Perfection and enter the Land of Good Enough using the GGB (Good-Better-Best) method (more discussion in CHAPTERS 5 AND 12). When we set ourselves up to work only in the Land of Perfection where only the BEST is acceptable, we jeopardize our chances of keeping the path to our goals open and clear. If you need to do fast food, order a salad and cut up a burger without the bun (or a grilled chicken) to put on top. If you can't drink all your water one day, just do your best to be hydrated with non-sugar beverages. If you are flat-out busy or exhausted and cannot go walking, do some ankle pumps and ankle circles to get the circulation going in your legs or just drop your head and try to reach the floor so you get a good stretch in. When you can do better, you will do better. But if you give up, then nothing gets done.

DO IT: Come on, just pick a day and start. It doesn't have to be a new week or a new month or even a new year. A fresh start can start with your next meal or the next choice you make between soda and water. Do it!

OWN IT: Don't do something because you want to please someone else. Do it because it's right for you and will make you happy and healthy. Make this *your* journey with *your* decisions and *your* actions. Own it!

WRITE IT DOWN: Don't have your goals dance around like little sugar plum fairies in your head. If you do that, then your goals will only be fairy tales and wishes. Work out your goal worksheet and pull out a calendar. Write it down!

NOW: Not tomorrow, not next week, not next year. You might have a delay on the start (you need to get those walking shoes and go grocery shopping for healthy food), but you do not have to delay thinking about, writing out and planning your goals. Take out a piece of paper and do it Now!

Before leaving the subject of setting goals, here is an example of the difference between a WHY and a GOAL. My first WHY was that I needed to bring down my blood sugar. My first GOAL in order to accomplish that WHY was to eat in a way where my blood sugar at night before bed would be no higher than 110. I further broke that goal down to things such as learning to use a nutrition tracker, dividing 20 total carbohydrates between three meals, adding fat to meals (in at least a 1.5:1 ratio, of fat to protein) so I would not be constantly hungry, not eating after dinner, etc. The WHY was general. The GOAL was specific in order to accomplish the WHY. The GOAL was Specific, Measurable, Achievable, Compatible, and I could keep up with the behaviors necessary to keep it going.

GOAL WORKSHEET

Write a goal. Any goal. Immediate or a long-term dream. You may have dozens of goals or you might have a burning goal that you want to tackle immediately. Start this practice sheet with the first one that comes to mind (it doesn't have to be weight loss!). Make several copies of the second sheet and work those goals until you reach your dreams.

WHAT IS MY GOAL:

S   Specific

M   Measurable

A   Achievable

C   Compatible

K   Keep it going

Are all criteria met so that the goal is workable and achievable?

NOW:

D   Do it (when?)

O   Own it (am I doing this for ME?)

W   Write it down (come on, don't just think it – ink it!)

N   **NOW**

What are the steps you need to do to get to the goal?

1.

2.

3.

4.

5.

6.

GOAL WORKSHEET

WHAT IS MY GOAL:

How do I make it:

S   Specific

M   Measurable

A   Achievable

C   Compatible

K   Keep it going

D   Do it

O   Own it

W   Write it down

N   **NOW**

What are the steps you need to do to get to the goal?

1.

2.

3.

4.

5.

6.

What are the steps I need to do to get to the goal?

1.

2.

3.

4.

5.

6.

CHAPTER TWENTY ONE

KAISEN

改善

Kaisen is a management system developed in Japan based on the idea that employees should be involved in continually improving products and services to make the company as successful as possible. I first heard of this concept from Tony Robbins, and I used it in my teaching from the moment I learned about it. I had very rigorous drills for my dancers that we did at the beginning of every class. I had some students who studied with me for years, decades even, and we never made big changes to the drills. To keep my students engaged in these drills I employed Kaisen. I asked them to improve their skills and performances by 1% a week. After a full semester they had improved by 20% or more. After a year or two they were 100% better than when they walked through my studio doors. Anyone can improve anything by 1%. The 1% builds on itself until you are far beyond your wildest dreams.

The SMACK DOWN method of goal setting is great, but it's still not enough. It is great to have the measurable and achievable goal of, let's say, walking first thing in the morning. But how will you do this? Here is part of the process, although you may choose a different order:

1. Lay my clothes out the night before.
2. I need to check the weather report.
3. I actually need new sneakers.
4. Go to the store and get new sneakers.
5. Find the time to go to the mall.
6. Ask partner to watch the kids while I go shopping.
7. Bring the right socks to try on sneakers.
8. ETC.

You can see it's all well and good to lay out your clothes but there is more to it than that. When you make your goals, make sure you look at all the steps you need to take to work on them. With this example, take the time to go to the mall, bring the right socks and find the time for yourself to go without the distraction of also watching your children. This is actually your first 1% – just finding time for yourself to do what you need to do to take care of yourself. Before going to bed you check the weather report to see if you need to wear shorts or pants or carry a light jacket with you in the morning. You never did this before. That is your next 1%. You get up 15 minutes earlier while your partner is still home to be with the kids, and you go for a short walk – your next 1%. Then you can increase your time/distance walking each day by another small percent. You can stay within that 15 minutes and increase your distance by percentages, you can increase your time by percentages, or both. In a month you are almost where you want to be. You are 100% better than you imagined that first day when you didn't even have sneakers or the right socks.

To accomplish this Kaisen, let's use Tony Robbins's *Massive Action Plan (MAP)*. This encompasses working with all the tools right in this section. First write down the results you want to achieve, then write down your compelling reason WHY you want to accomplish your goals. Finally develop a sequence of actions and steps to achieve this. Here is an example of my MAP, which also incorporates Kaisen. This means that some steps are "stand-alone," but some steps build upon one another.

This is a suggestion of how to set up a MAP that incorporates *Granny Keto Transitions Program*™ so that you can relate it to what your goals might be in this process. Use the same process for your MAP.

RESULT: The sugar monkey is off my back. I am free.

WHY: I am sick of overeating sugar and baked goods and feeling I can't live without them.

STEPS:

1. Thoroughly read *Granny Keto Transitions Program*™, Step 1. (CHAPTER 3)

2. Go through my pantry and fridge take stock of all the foods with sugar and flour.

3. Get rid of what my family won't miss.

4. If room allows, put sugar desserts, breads, chips, etc. in a separate spot, preferably in a cabinet or basket where I won't see them all the time.

5. Sit down with my family, even the little kids, and explain that I am going to cut out sugar and other treats so that I will be healthy. Ask them to please honor and respect what I am doing because we all love one another, and that from now on their treats will be in a special spot just for them. Further explain that I am not asking them to cut anything out. Right now, it is just for me.

6. Go to the meal planning worksheets and see how I can make dinners that will eliminate things like pasta and bread for me but can be served on the side for the family.

7. Go to the packing lunches worksheet to see what I can take for my lunches.

8. Go to the Grocery Shopping worksheet and make a list.

9. Each evening write out a Protocol meal plan (or something specific if that is what I want to do) as a road map for the next day so I can make sure I know what I am eating. Doing a couple in advance is even better so I make sure I have the food I need.

10. Try my best to do a mindfulness practice at least once a day.

11. No need to write a full journal. Just write down on my meal plan page what my accomplishment was for the day.

Chapter Twenty Two

Circumstance-Thoughts-Feelings-Actions-Results

(CTFAR)

This is a concept that many successful people use. I first learned about it from working with Brooke Castillo at her Life Coach School. She refers to it as *The Model*. "Always work the model," she says. This is a very valuable tool in your toolbox. We often hear the term *mindset* and how it is important to everything we do. CTFAR (Circumstances, Thoughts, Feelings, Actions, and Results) are the gears and workings of your mindset. The process of working this model will help you break down the thoughts that cause your feelings, which dictate your actions that lead to your results. We often blame our circumstances for the difficulties in our life, but it is really our thoughts *about* our circumstances that dictate our results. In order to change the results of your life you need to change your thoughts. This is the ultimate way to change how we feel and behave. Be in charge of how you think.

Here is the model is and how to work it.

Circumstance: These are **unarguable** facts that describe a situation, not your thoughts or feelings about the situation. For example: It is June 1. I weigh 200 pounds. The dress I have in my closet does not fit. I go walking every day.

Thoughts: These can be **arguable** and unique to your own brain. For instance: It is a crappy day (someone else: I love these kinds of days – overcast and chilly). I am so fat at 200 pounds (someone else: I would love to be only 200 pounds – wouldn't that be terrific?). The dress I have looks awful and I need a new dress (someone else: The dress I have might not fit perfectly but if I wear a scarf or shawl, it will cover the flaws and I will look gorgeous). I go walking every day but it's a crappy day for walking today (someone else: I could use a break. I will do an exercise video instead).

Can you see the difference between thought and circumstance? A circumstance is the same no matter who is looking at it. Circumstances are facts. Thoughts take those circumstances and put your own personal spin on them. You might think something is a fact such as "It's a crappy day" but indeed, someone else might think it is a beautiful day. That's a THOUGHT, not a FACT. The most successful way to work a model is to, right from the start, learn what it means to be a circumstance and what it means to be a thought.

Feelings: A feeling is how you feel about the thought, and that's why it comes next. For instance, the fact is that it is June 1. Your thought about it is that it is a crappy day. Your feeling about it is that such a day makes you FEEL depressed. When you say "I'm depressed" that is how a certain thought about a certain fact makes you feel. You cannot expect everyone to feel the same way you do, but, alas, you do. "What do you mean you're happy?" "What do you mean you love this kind of weather?" "What do you mean these are your most productive days when you get the most done?" Usually when you have tacked a feeling onto a thought, you have dug yourself deep into a trench. A lot of people say they can't help how they feel. But really, they can. The problem with the difficulty in changing a feeling is that you think it is a fact. It is not. From these feelings (good, bad or indifferent) flow your actions.

Actions: An action is what you do in response to your feelings. Let's take that crappy day again. Because you think the weather is crappy, you feel depressed and miserable about it. There are many actions you might employ because you feel depressed and miserable. Maybe you won't even want to get out of bed and "face the day." Maybe you will begrudgingly get out of bed and do the minimal self-care because being depressed has zapped the energy out of you. Maybe you will get your work done for the day, but half-heartedly. Forget exercise. I bet some of you who go faithfully to the gym know when you are having an "off" day and the workout just does not feel satisfying. And forget about dieting – who the heck wants to diet in crappy weather? (You can exercise and diet, but you know what I am talking about!) These are some of the actions that spring from the feeling that you are depressed because of the thought that it is a crappy day, when the only circumstance here is that it is June 1.

Results: Let's take a look at the results that flow from these actions. IF you manage to get out of bed, you didn't take care of yourself. All day your hair isn't at its best. Your clothes may be mussed or ill-fitting. Maybe you didn't have a good breakfast or, heaven forbid, didn't stop for coffee. You might also have skipped your workout or had an unproductive one and, OMG you had a fender-bender. Do you think you had a good dinner? I think not! Ultimate result: You don't feel good about your choices or actions. If one day turns into two, and two into three (regardless of the weather because now your actions-results take on a life of their own), you are lamenting about how you "fell off the wagon" and can't find your footing again.

Let's look at the models for some of these circumstances, following through to the actions and results. The first column is the "unintentional" model, meaning these are the thoughts and feelings that flow from your perception of the circumstance. The actions and results flow from your thoughts and feelings. The second column takes the same circumstances but asks you to intentionally pick better (or alternative) thoughts and feelings. You will see that more productive actions and results flow from the "intentional" model.

UNINTENTIONAL MODEL	INTENTIONAL MODEL
C: It is June 1.	C: It is June 1.
T: It's a crappy day.	T: It's just a day. It's only rain.
F: I'm depressed.	F: Any day above ground is a good day!
A: I lay around all day.	A: I get up and take care of myself.
R: Another wasted day.	R: I get things done and feel good.
C: I weigh 200 pounds.	C: I weigh 200 pounds.
T: I'm so fat.	T: It's just a number.
F: I am not worth "it."	F: I am more than this and worth it.
A: I eat junk to feel better.	A: I stay on plan and push through.
R: I stay fat and miserable.	R: I have lost weight!
C: My dress does not fit.	C: My dress does not fit.
T: The dress looks awful.	T: It's a nice dress.
F: I 'll never look good.	F: I usually feel great in this dress.
A: I eat to feel better.	A: I can add a shawl to cover it up a bit.
R: I stay fat and miserable.	R: I am motivated to lose a little more weight.
C: I go walking for exercise.	C: I go walking for exercise.
T: It's all I'm good at.	T: I can try new things.
F: I hate doing anything else.	F: I might find something else I like.
A: I don't walk in bad weather.	A: I can do exercise videos on a bad day.
R: I stay fat and miserable.	R: I fit into the dress without a shawl!

CTFAR WORKSHEET

Try your own CTFAR (Circumstances, Thoughts, Feelings, Actions, and Results). For right now, just pick one or two things. Work out whether they are circumstance, thoughts or feelings. Then work out the actions and results. Sometimes in confusing a thought for a circumstance, people might confuse action with results. Pay attention to what you are putting in each line, then step back and ask yourself if everything you put down is in the correct category. If a model needs changes in thoughts or feelings, or actions and results, write the same circumstance but work it differently like I did in my sample Intentional Model. Use this page to practice right now. Then you can either copy the second worksheet page, get a small notebook or set of index cards and hand write CTFAR on each.

UNINTENTIONAL MODEL	INTENTIONAL MODEL
C:	C:
T:	T:
F:	F:
A:	A:
R:	R:

UNINTENTIONAL MODEL	INTENTIONAL MODEL
C:	C:
T:	T:
F:	F:
A:	A:
R:	R:

UNINTENTIONAL MODEL	INTENTIONAL MODEL
C:	C:
T:	T:
F:	F:
A:	A:
R:	R:

UNINTENTIONAL MODEL	INTENTIONAL MODEL
C:	C:
T:	T:
F:	F:
A:	A:
R:	R:

UNINTENTIONAL MODEL	INTENTIONAL MODEL
C:	C:
T:	T:
F:	F:
A:	A:
R:	R:

UNINTENTIONAL MODEL	INTENTIONAL MODEL
C:	C:
T:	T:
F:	F:
A:	A:
R:	R:

UNINTENTIONAL MODEL	INTENTIONAL MODEL
C:	C:
T:	T:
F:	F:
A:	A:
R:	R:

CHAPTER TWENTY THREE

RECOGNIZING AND SITTING WITH URGES

An urge is a strong desire or impulse. *The urge to eat is just a thought.* An urge is most likely a response to some sort of trigger. The trigger could be physical (you smell fresh bread, and you want it immediately), emotional (you need a distraction from a thought or a chore) or it could be habit (you always eat while watching TV at night).

When we dieters fall headlong into an urge no matter how "hard" we are trying to stay on plan, we think we are stupid, lazy or broken. We feel we are damaged goods and will never lose weight. What we don't realize is that we are actually *brilliant*! We are acting on patterns that have always served us in the past. We don't have to do any thinking because we are brilliantly on autopilot. The trick is to stop the autopilot and give these thoughts and actions the attention they deserve.

Remember that there is nothing wrong with you. With an emotional trigger, for instance, you have a pattern of turning to food when you don't want to face things. The food might not be anything more than a distraction. It may be a repeated pattern of immediate gratification. It may be a pattern of using food to feel better in the moment. You are not broken or hopeless because you give in to urges. You just have to learn to reframe your response to circumstances. My "Stop, Drop and Roll" worksheet at the end of this chapter will help you with this reframing.

The first step is to acknowledge the urge, identify its trigger and ask yourself whether that trigger is true (are the kids really *devils* or are they doing what kids *normally* do?) and whether the food we seek will actually solve the problem.

What do you do in urge territory? In the immediate, just sit and breathe. Don't do too much thinking. Set a timer if you have one on hand. Sometimes sitting with the urge for two to three minutes will help you get past it. Sometimes it takes much longer to get your mind off of it. Close your eyes. Breathe slowly.

What? You don't have time to sit and breathe? You have time to go to the store and purchase candy. You have time to go out to eat it in the car and then drive home. But you don't have time to sit and breathe for a few minutes? Come on.

Sometimes if you busy yourself with a task, that will help. Write in a journal. Turn on the TV and sit on your hands. Do a "Stop, Drop and Roll" worksheet. For sure, get out of the kitchen if you are home. If it is a simple trigger urge, get out of the bakery section of the supermarket or drink a bottle of water while your kids are having ice cream. You can *always* interrupt an urge if you are inclined to do so.

What do you do when you find that you cannot get out of urge territory, when it is deeper than the smell of freshly baked bread or the desire to avoid a task? This is where you have to do some introspection and reflection. This is where you have to examine your WHY (CHAPTER 19) and decide if reaching your goal is, or is not, more important than that candy or bread or ice cream. Again, understand that **nothing is wrong with you**. You have a *pattern* of turning to food when you don't want to face things. Eating the food can be a simple distraction, such as having a snack instead of folding laundry. Sometimes eating the food can be a little more than "just" a distraction. It might serve a deeper purpose. For instance, once you have finished the binge you are so busy beating yourself up about it and may be feeling sick, that you have no room in your brain to think of the fight you just had with a friend. It may be a *pattern* of immediate gratification or a *pattern* of using food to feel better in the moment. And sometimes, a pattern is just a pattern. A pattern for me used to be the urge to finish the mac and cheese from my grandson's bowl. I still might have the urge, but I now see it for what it is: merely a pattern. I easily throw it away or cover it for his snack later.

I want to digress for a moment with a story, but it makes the point of turning to food for comfort. When my daughter was around six, she fell and hurt herself. I gave her a cookie and told her it would make her feel better. She looked at me very puzzled, and while she was asking why it would make her feel better, she put it on her knee where she hurt herself. If I had answered, "No, eat it. THAT will make you feel better," I would have raised a daughter who turns to food for *any* sort of comfort. Now, as an adult, she won't even eat if she's hungry and dinner is less than an hour away. How did a girl like this spring from the loins of a person who has had food issues since *her* age of six?

Some of the work here is in recognizing cravings vs. urges. Urges will bury you unless you face them. The very first thing you need to do is to stop and ask yourself if you are hungry. Plain and simple. Identify the number. If you are under a 5 then eat, and not necessarily the urge food. You may have felt the urge because your stomach's bells and whistles were going off. You still can, and should, eat sensibly. If you are at a 5 or above, then chances are you are in pure urge territory (nothing to do with hunger).

If you need to, please go back to THE HUNGER SCALE (CHAPTER 12 and the Mindfulness Practice in CHAPTER 6) each and every time you *think* you feel hungry and also at the beginning and end of every meal. Once you know yourself and find that you are 5 or below on the scale, go ahead and eat. You are hungry! You might be craving something, but that is still different from an urge.

To address cravings: Even with a craving such as pizza and beer, Chinese food or whatever, if you have mastered where you are on the hunger scale (to know if you are truly hungry and when you have had enough), even a craving won't be enough to sidetrack you. Once you have learned when you are satisfied (6) or can stop yourself mid-way through a 7 (full) before you have done any damage, physically or emotionally, you can address cravings with little worry. In other words, if you are craving pizza and (1) it is allowed on whichever food program you are following, and (2) you have identified you are hungry and later when you are full – even if that means leaving some behind or having a little bit more, it will make no difference whether you have eaten the pizza or a salad with tuna on top. With this example, and you are eating low carb and only eat between a 4 and a 6, then this is where there might be little difference between the salad and the pizza. As long as you do not overeat and you are aware of your carbohydrate intake the rest of the day, your choice may not make a difference. If you are on a keto food plan, then no, you won't want to have the pizza (unless you have made a keto crust). You will have to sit with that craving a bit and go back to your WHY, just as you do with an urge.

Whether you are dealing with urges or cravings please understand, and therefore I repeat, you are not damaged goods, stupid, lazy or broken. You have to interrupt the pattern that you have so *brilliantly* learned. Up until now you have practiced and integrated your urge response into your everyday behavior. Once you realize this and do the physical things to stop the urge from progressing, you will start to feel better about yourself. You will always have urges. They won't disappear. What will change is your reaction to them. Just put a little space between the urge and the giving in to that urge, and pretty soon that space will get longer and longer until you can just go on with your day.

URGE WORKSHEET: STOP, DROP AND ROLL

Remember: An urge is just a thought! Let's go back to the CTFAR (Circumstances, Thoughts, Feelings, Actions, and Results) exercise for this. Let's put out that fire!

WHAT YOU ARE EXPERIENCING:	LET'S FLIP THIS ON ITS HEAD:
C: I want ice cream	C: I want ice cream.
T: It is calling my name.	T: It is not calling my name. I'm not hungry and I don't need it.
F: I deserve it.	F: I deserve to feel good about being able to sit with this urge for a few minutes.
A: I will go into the kitchen and get it.	A: I am going to put away laundry instead.
R: Yet again, I feel broken and stupid, and I think I will never get this right.	R: Great! I did it! The urge passed. I can do this!

Another urge:

WHAT YOU ARE EXPERIENCING:	**LET'S FLIP THIS ON ITS HEAD:**
C: I want cookies.	C: I want cookies.
T: I've been so good all day. I should reward myself.	T: I've been good all day but I'm not a dog. I don't need a reward.
F: One or two won't hurt me.	F: I will feel better about myself if I don't have even one or two.
A: I don't stop at one or two. I eat the sleeve.	A: I turn off the light and leave the kitchen.
R: Yet again, I feel broken and stupid, and I won't even bother tomorrow.	R: Yay! I lost a pound this week AND feel great about myself.

YOUR STOP, DROP AND ROLL WORKSHEET

What are you thinking right now?

C:

T:

F:

A:

R:

How can you turn this around?

C:

T:

F:

A:

R:

_____

What are you thinking right now?

C:

T:

F:

A:

R:

How can you turn this around?

C:

T:

F:

A:

R:

Chapter Twenty Four

Self-Talk

In my book, *Language of the Dance – Belly Dance with Amira Jamal,* I have a worksheet entitled STOP THAT NEGATIVE SELF-TALK. It was one of the most important – and popular – lessons in my classes. It is probably one of the most important things you need to learn to have a successful journey with *whatever* you are doing.

Self-talk is your inner voice. It is what you are telling yourself all day long as your day unfolds. It can be positive, giving you confidence, encouragement, compliments, optimism, direction and motivation. It can be negative, fostering discouragement, pointing out your faults and shortcomings, giving you the pessimistic side of things, totally derailing any hopes, dreams and goals you may have. It is not unusual or uncommon to have some of your thoughts be negative. There is research, or at least speculation, that we have tens of thousands of thoughts per day. Some are in a continuous loop and some are random or in reaction to something specific. No matter the number, they cannot be expected to be all positive and wonderful. However, there is no reason to make them all negative and awful either. Negative self-talk is not helpful. As matter of fact, it can be damaging not only to our self-esteem, but it may cause some of us to turn to food which is exactly what we are trying to change. When you have a negative thought stop and ask yourself, "Is this true?"

Talk to yourself the way you would to a friend. Be kind and have compassion. A friend comes to you and says, "I am so stupid and lazy. I am trying to follow *Granny Keto Transitions Program*™ and I can't even get through Step 1. Every morning I wake up and say I am not going to have sugar today. By the time my head hits the pillow I have "blown it" again. Stupid, stupid, stupid." Okay, so you are this person's friend. Are you going to say, "Yes, you really are stupid and lazy. You are worthless. Don't even bother..."? Or are you going to say, "This is a really big life change that involves a lot of steps to see it through. Maybe you have to break it up into even smaller steps than you have been doing. How about having a water bottle or even some gum handy, and the next time you want that cookie, reach for the alternative. Better yet, put a pack of gum and a small water bottle where you keep the cookies for the kids. Stop and count to ten and decide which one to reach for. Each and every time you don't put something sweet in your mouth, stop and compliment yourself. Realize you have taken a big step. Be kind to yourself. You are not a loser, and you are not lazy. Just the fact that you are looking for a better life shows that you are not lazy." Now, imagine that you are that friend. Speak kindly to yourself. Speak positively to yourself. Speak encouragingly to yourself. Mother Theresa said, "Kind words can be short and easy to speak, but their echoes are truly endless." You don't have to have long speeches with yourself. When your hand shoots back from the cookies and picks up the gum just say, "Good job!"

Furthermore, nothing good ever comes of hatred. Some of you might really hate yourselves, either because of your weight or your inability to follow through with a goal. Indulge me with another Mother Theresa quote: "I will never attend an anti-war rally; if you have a peace rally, invite me." Drop the negative self-talk as much as you can and have a peace rally with yourself: "You can do this. You are smart and capable. You just haven't figured it out yet. That little step of reaching for the gum instead of the cookie was a great accomplishment. I've got your back. I love you." Be kind.

SELF-TALK WORKSHEET

Catch your thinking and self-talk as much as you can. If you catch yourself thinking something like, "Idiot. You just ate that cookie," counter it with, "You have turned to food all your life either mindlessly to avoid something or to feel better. You are not an idiot. You are doing what you know to do. That's actually pretty smart! BUT – it's time to learn to do something new. I love you."

Here is a worksheet with some thoughts related to eating. Use the blank worksheet on the following page for yourself. Make it a dedicated "exercise" or just jot down your thoughts when you are aware of them.

NEGATIVE THOUGHTS	POSITIVE REPLACEMENTS
I'm so lazy I don't even go for a walk.	Start with just walking around the block. I bet after you are walking for a little while you will look forward to longer walks.
I'm so stupid. I was "good" all day and ate a box of cookies before going to bed.	Well, you are not stupid. You are usually tired and anxious by the end of the day, very fertile conditions for overeating. Tomorrow night just stop and try to sit with your anxiety a few minutes and also try to go to bed a little earlier if you can.
I can't do this.	Yes, you can. There is a lot that is going well. You have been making meal plans – maybe you just have to make them more realistic so that they are easier to follow. AND you passed that box of cookies in the grocery store today! Good job!

Your positive replacements can become your new affirmations! Talk to yourself in the mirror!

STOP THAT NEGATIVE SELF-TALK WORKSHEET

Negative Thoughts	Positive Replacements

Chapter Twenty Five

Mindfulness Practices

A lot of us get into trouble because we are not mindful when we are eating. How many of us have looked at an empty plate, an empty chip bag or empty cookie box and have said, "Where did that go?" Go back to the mindfulness practices in each of the *Granny Keto Transitions Program*™ steps to review and practice them. Below are some more practices, but I also encourage you to find some of your own. A lot of these practices are perfect opportunities to set up a Kaisen practice. For instance, your goal might be to sit at the table while you are eating. However, you might need several steps to get there.

- You'll stop eating in the car.
- You'll stop eating standing up at the counter or in front of the fridge.
- Move to the table with the bag of chips.
- How about eating snacks from a bowl?
- Then put the snacks in a large bowl, then a medium one, then a small one.
- How about setting out a napkin?

You might need all these steps to reach your mindfulness practice goal of sitting at the table with your food. Each step is an improvement over the one before. Don't discount the small steps. Here are the mindfulness practices for each step of *Granny Keto Transitions Program*™:

- Put down your fork after every bite. (CHAPTER 3)
- Ask: What do I want? What do I need? What do I have? (CHAPTER 4)
- Pay attention to how a particular food makes you feel. (CHAPTER 5)
- Learn your hunger scale. (CHAPTER 6)
- Slow down: Chew slowly, swallow, breathe. (CHAPTER 7)

What are some mindfulness practices you can think of, or which of these would you like to work on? Practice developing your own mindful practices and use the worksheet to examine the practices you would like to work on and steps you will need. Here are a few more to get you practicing!

- Sit at the table when you eat.
- Have gratitude for your meal.
- Eliminate distractions. Just eat.
- Bring other senses to the table like smell and sight.

- No judgment. If you are eating cake, enjoy every bite!
- Practice positive self-talk.
- Practice positive affirmations.
- Recognize when you have stopped an urge or craving.
- Recognize and congratulate yourself for NSVs (non-scale victories).
- Recognize and congratulate yourself for bringing Kaisen into your life.

Mindfulness Practice	Am I able to do it right now? YES? DO IT! NO? Work on next column.	What steps do I need to take (as in the chip example above)?

MINDFULNESS PRACTICE WORKSHEET

Mindfulness Practice	Am I able to do it right now? YES? DO IT! NO? Work on next column.	What steps do I need to take (as in the chip example above)?

Mindfulness Practice	Am I able to do it right now? YES? DO IT! NO? Work on next column.	What steps do I need to take (as in the chip example above)?

Mindfulness Practice	Am I able to do it right now? YES? DO IT! NO? Work on next column.	What steps do I need to take (as in the chip example above)?

Chapter Twenty Six

Your Relationship with Yourself

I saved this chapter for last because it is not your relationship with food that determines if you can stick to a program (*any* program), lose weight or accomplish any of your non-food goals. It is your relationship with yourself that determines any and all success that you have. This last chapter was the hardest for me to write. I stopped and started it several times. Forgive me in advance for all the sayings and corny metaphors, but certain words become sayings and metaphors for a reason. Here goes…

I wanted to convey that you are capable of reaching your dreams, but you also have to understand that nothing is linear. As you travel up and down and hit all the speed bumps, detours and forks in the road, you need to learn to go with the flow. Let's say you come out in the morning and have a flat tire. Sure, you are mad and maybe even blame yourself for driving over a nail. But the point is, you don't go slash the other three. You fix the one. Because you may have finished a whole pizza at lunch does not mean you stop trying. It means that you start again at the next meal. You start as many times as you need to. Realize that you are doing things from old patterns. You are not stupid or broken. You can't grow new plants from old seeds. Disrupt the soil and plant some new seeds.

As my good friend, Amy Smith, reminded me the other day, "The universe is unfolding as it should." As I was sitting at my computer last night, I was wondering how I would sum up the crux of what I want to share with you. You can get any and all information about keto and low carb ways of eating from the Internet, dozens of books, hundreds of cookbooks and thousands of YouTube videos. But I need to teach you something that, if you don't get it, no amount of instruction will help you succeed. The story is: I had a run-in with a family brunch this morning and apparently that is how my universe perfectly unfolded so that I could finish this book.

Even if you don't see it or don't believe it now, you *are* capable of success. You *are* smart. You *are* worthwhile. What happened that was the perfect timing for writing this chapter? This morning, for the first time in three months, since the beginning of COVID 19, I had my daughter and son-in-law and two grandchildren over for Sunday brunch. No face masks. Hugging. The whole shebang. I prepared my usual brunch foods (muffins, bagels, etc.) along with a lovely array of keto foods (smoked salmon/cream cheese rollups, salami, olives, eggs, etc.). I ate all the keto foods. I was at least at a 6 on the hunger scale. Then I ate a muffin and a bagel. I would have had more except that I was easily at a 7 or 8 at this point. There was nothing else I really wanted, and I knew enough to not make myself sick by getting to a 9 or 10.

So there. The author of this book is telling you to sit with urges, honor your hunger scale, examine your WHY, stick to it, etc. etc., and here she polished off a muffin (granted just a quarter of one but that's not the point) and a full bagel with cream cheese. Oh, and she finished her granddaughter's half bagel with butter. There may have been a cookie involved. There. I did it. But I am not going to erase this entire book, hate myself and never try again.

What I am going to do is probably feel sorry for myself as I pop a TUMS®, after which I will go to Staples® and run out a draft of this book so that I can sit with a red pen and edit. I am going to realize that I am intelligent and worthwhile. I am going to realize that I wasn't even approaching the Land of Good Enough as I plowed through that bagel. I am going to understand that I still have something to offer, maybe even more so. What I am *not* going to do is continue to eat all day until I am sick. I am *not* going to beat myself up until I feel so unworthy that I will never want to publish this book. I am *not* going to throw in the towel and throw out what I know is the best way of eating for me. Instead, I am going to sit for a minute and reflect. I am going to see what lessons might come out of this. The lesson is not to be afraid to serve anything and everything, but to really put in that "speed bump" I wrote about. Put a pause between wanting the food and eating the food. The lesson, perhaps, is to remove myself from the table. There is always something to do in the kitchen even though I have company. Believe me everyone is so busy eating they never even would notice if I got up!

More importantly I need to acknowledge, with no hateful emotions, that I ate what I ate, and I am worthy of moving on.

Throughout this book I wanted to know exactly where to share the Buddha's parable of *The Second Arrow*, and this is it. The story goes as follows: A person is walking through a forest and gets struck by an arrow, which causes great pain. He asks, "Should I stay here and let myself get struck by another arrow?" The first arrow is the circumstance, which we often cannot control. The second arrow is our reaction to it. We often hear that "Pain is inevitable, suffering is optional." If you get struck by an arrow, do you then shoot another arrow into yourself or allow others to?

This is what happens over and over and over again when we are following a food plan, "fall off the wagon," and then continue to shoot one arrow after another into our hearts and souls. The second arrows come with the messages: "I'm stupid," "I'm not good enough," "I'll never get this right," "This is too hard," "I'm too lazy," "I'm not worthwhile," "I hate myself." STOP IT WITH THE SECOND ARROWS! No matter how perfectly you follow a food plan, you are, at one time or another going to get struck with that first arrow – maybe many different times. It's painful. Get up, move on and don't suffer. Learn your lessons and be grateful for what you have learned so far.

Good luck. I love you. We can do this together.

Appendix

More Ways of Making Keto a Lifestyle

Here are some other popular ways to do keto in addition to the two ways suggested in Chapter 10, Ways of Doing Keto, eating from a "Yes/No" list and counting Macros.

Lazy Keto

"Lazy Keto" is, in a nutshell, keeping your carbohydrates to 20 grams or less, total or net, and just eating from Yes/No lists. There is nothing wrong with this if you combine it with your hunger and satiety signals. However, it can often turn into a free-for-all even though what you are eating comes from a Yes/No list. In this case, a person is likely to eat protein and fat past satiety, which will result in too much food for the body's needs, resulting in fat storage. As I have already said, just changing your way of eating from the Standard American Diet to keto (or low carb) will result in an initial weight loss and internal healing. Sometimes continuing along this Lazy Keto route may result in hitting a wall, so to speak. If you really put the time into learning your body's signals (eat when hungry – stop when full) you may never see that wall, let alone hit it. Work on, and overcome, any mindless habits, along with honoring your hunger and fullness scale, to make this a wonderfully successful method.

IIFYM

IIFYM stands for If It Fits Your Macros. It is sometimes called "Dirty Keto." As with Lazy Keto, a person following this way of eating will initially experience weight loss. However, there will not always be internal healing. People who do IIFYM eat low enough carbohydrates to call it keto because they are producing ketones. However, true keto healing includes lowering inflammation in the body and not just being able to produce ketones. A lot of inflammation comes from the ingestion of sugar, wheat and grain products, which many people following IIFYM will eat. Keto dictates the type of foods that are eaten, not just the carbohydrate counts, so IIFYM is potentially not a true keto diet.

Dairy-Free

Butter and ghee are up for discussion in the dairy-free camp. Both are made from milk. However, they are both considered fat rather than protein. Ghee is lactose-free because all of the milk solids are completely removed during production and butter contains only trace amounts of lactose. If you are avoiding dairy because you are lactose-intolerant, these are usually safe fat options for you, although they are not dairy-free. But why do people decide to go dairy-free at all? A large percentage of the population is sensitive to dairy. There are two components to dairy that could be the culprits: either the lactose (sugar) or casein (protein). However, overall, even if you do not have a dairy sensitivity, dairy is a known inflammatory and many people choose to cut it out altogether.

CARNIVORE

Carnivore is eating only animal products and fat. There are few plant products, if at all (usually, olives, olive oil, avocados and avocado oil). People who follow this way of eating do not count anything – they just eat and enjoy! Eating the fat and protein is self-limiting when you tune in to your hunger cues. There are people who have found tremendous health benefits eating this way. I am not looking to defend or deny the virtues of the carnivore way of eating keto, but there are a few questions that often come up in a carnivore discussion. They are: Will I become constipated? Do I risk kidney damage? Am I getting enough vitamins? The short answers are NO, NO and YES, respectively. The full answers are in CHAPTER 11, QUESTIONS AND DISPELLING MYTHS.

Eating carnivore, with or without dairy, is growing in popularity and I strongly urge you to do your own research. Many people enjoy carnivore and do well with it. Others do not feel well and find that adding back vegetables helps them immensely. It may have to do with your DNA or gut microbiome. Vegetables and certain nuts and seeds also deliver estrogen and phytoestrogen which are very important, especially for women. Do what is best for you and not what the latest post on social media tells you to do. This is where listening to your body, in addition to hunger and fullness signals, is invaluable.

One last thing: Do not use this way of eating as punishment or a way to manipulate yourself. Carnivore even further restricts eating choices and sometimes a person would do this but not see it as punishment for not losing weight fast enough or as a punishment for a binge or going off their keto food plan. Go into this plan from a place of curiosity to see if it will improve your overall health and not as punishment for being "bad."

FASTING AND EATING WINDOWS

Fasting has, of late, become the buzz word in all the diet magazines and morning talk shows. Nothing new about fasting! It has been around for centuries as part of religious practices or even since caveman days when it could be days between hunts for fresh food. But fast-forward to this century, and specifically this decade, and it has become a tool in many diet regimens. With keto it is usually not a total fast (i.e., you drink water and take electrolyte supplementation and thus do not risk dehydration). You may hear the terms EF and IF. These stand for **Extended Fasting** and **Intermittent Fasting**.

Intermittent Fasting (IF) could be 24 hours or less (with eating windows of 2 to 12 hours). Most people achieve this either with OMAD (described below) or setting a more generous eating window with more than one meal. These windows are most commonly 12:12, 16:8, 20:4, and 22:2. A time of 12:12 means you fast for 12 hours and eat your meals within the other 12, and 16:8 means you fast for 16 and eat within the remaining 8. The hours 20:4 means you fast for 20 hours and eat within the remaining 4, and 22:2 means you fast for 22 hours and eat within the remaining 2 (the usual structure for OMAD). Another way to accomplish IF is to fast for 24 hours once or twice a week. The combinations are many and varied.

Under no circumstances should you do an Extended Fast without guidance and permission from your doctor, especially if you are on medication, and specifically if you are on diabetes medication. I think what upset me the most about various Facebook groups is when there is a fasting challenge done online. I often see groups get together with "Let's do a five-day fast! Who's with me?" and the results can be harmful. I recall a woman nearly dying because she did this without supervision, came off her diabetes medication without consulting her doctor, and her glucose numbers were crazy off the wall – both high and low. Yet, at the beginning everyone was cheering her on because she did the fast and came off the medication herself without a doctor's approval. I see these challenges in various groups weekly (sometimes daily) and it breaks my heart that people are so desperate for high ketone readings and faster weight loss that they will foolishly do these things. Don't throw out the baby with the bathwater. It is not the fault of keto or fasting. It is the fault of ignorantly enthusiastic people who happen to be doing keto.

FAT FASTING

With fasting, either IF or EF, some people will consume less than 500 calories, most likely in fat. This is different from *fat fasting*, which is a program offered by IDM, Intensive Dietary Management (Jason Fung). This is the outline given by Megan Ramos of IDM for fat fasting:

1. Eat when hungry, until full, as often as necessary.

2. Do not have dairy or nuts during a fat fast.

3. You may use up to three tablespoons (daily) of heavy cream for your tea or coffee.

4. You may consume eggs, bacon, salmon, sardines, olive oil, coconut oil, MCT oil, avocado oil, macadamia nut oil, butter, ghee, mayo (healthy oil base), avocado, olives, leafy greens cooked in or covered in fat, bone broth, tea and coffee. You may also use spices.

5. Leafy greens cooked in, or covered in, fat.

6. Bone broth, coffee and tea.

No matter which fasting pattern you choose, almost everyone will say "Eat if you are hungry," except for the crazy group that encouraged that poor woman to keep going.

OMAD

OMAD stands for One Meal a Day. It is a type of intermittent fasting and it is just what it sounds like. However, as with IIFYM (If It Fits Your Macros), many people eat foods that are not at all keto (such as lasagna, bread sticks and a hefty dessert). In the keto version of OMAD, you would eat only keto foods but would consume them at one large meal. Many people find success with this way of eating, but others find that they cannot meet the nutritional needs of their bodies unless they truly gorge on fats and protein. One successful way to do this, however, is to take a one to two hour eating window so that you break your day's fast with something light like a soup or a salad. Then eat the main meal and perhaps finish with some berries and beverage with heavy cream. This doesn't give the same feeling as eating a lot in a short amount of time and allows those calories and nutrients to be eaten in a more leisurely way. The one meal can be breakfast, lunch or dinner. As with IIFYM, this has the potential to become a free-for-all diet unless only keto foods are consumed during your one meal.

A true OMAD style suggests drinking only black coffee or tea, water or sparkling water all day until the one meal is consumed. This is suggested to assure there will be no insulin response coming from any other source than the one meal. There is one school of thought that says that because there is little to no insulin response from fat, that up to 500 fat calories can be consumed without affecting the OMAD success. I personally have to chuckle to think this might have been written by a coffee addict who needed her cream. It is worth noting here that sweeteners can cause an insulin response for some people and should also be avoided if you are doing OMAD.

KETO FOR ATHLETES

This is a way of eating where the protein is scaled way up beyond the usual suggested limits. This may be fine if you are looking to build serious muscle, as in training for a body-building championship, but is not needed for normal wear-and-tear exercise. Even an hour in the gym every day or training for a marathon will not increase your need for protein as much as some of these groups would have you believe. If you are a dedicated athlete do your homework.

CARB CYCLING

This is an approach where you eat a higher amount of carbohydrates on either a regular basis (once a week, every other day, etc.) or as needed. For instance, many women find some relief if they add extra carbohydrates during their menstrual cycles. Increase carbohydrates through natural whole foods such as adding a sweet potato or other root vegetables to a meal. Carb cycling does not give you permission to eat candy bars and chocolate cake once a week! There has also been some anecdotal evidence that carb cycling may increase your body's ability to burn fat in the long run by making your body metabolically flexible. People who are very keen on this method of keto are Leanne Vogel, Dr. Will Cole and Mark Sisson. I recommend that you do some research on the purported benefits of carb cycling if you are interested. If you are severely insulin resistant or have other metabolic issues, this might not be for you. Do your research. Remember: It does not mean you have permission to pig out once a week – even if you schedule it into your food plan.

RESOURCES

Podcasts and websites and cookbooks, oh my! In addition to all the books and studies that I read when I started keto, some podcasts and websites were invaluable. You can Google both and find hundreds, but these are the ones that were precious to me in my education about all things keto – from science to cooking!

PODCASTS

There are many informative podcasts on following a keto lifestyle. When I commuted to work, I spent 3-4 hours a day in the car if it was a bad traffic day. I never minded it at all. I knew all the bathrooms along the route, and I had my podcasts. To get you started, I am listing my top ten choices for learning about low carb and keto, although over the years I have listened to many more wonderful ones. A great deal of what I learned about keto in the beginning came from these podcasts. Some are no longer podcasting, but they are still available through various podcast subscription sites.

- Livin' La Vida Low Carb with Jimmy Moore
- Keto Talk with Jimmy Moore and Adam Nally
- 2 Keto Dudes with Richard Morris and Carl Franklin
- The Obesity Code Podcast with Jason Fung and Megan Ramos
- Keto Woman Podcast with Daisy Brackenhall
- What the Fat with Dr. Ryan Lowery
- Real Talk with Jimmy Moore and Will Cole
- Diet Doctor with Bret Scher
- The Keto Happy Hour with Emily Pierce
- The Keto Answers Podcast with Dr. Anthony Gustin

WEBSITES

As with podcasts, and maybe more so, there are hundreds of websites devoted to low carb and keto. If you add all the recipe websites devoted to both, you maybe have thousands to choose from. In this list below, I am giving you some of my favorites that provide educational material and resources about these ways of eating. Some sell their products, although sales are not at the forefront of what they offer on their websites. I included only a couple of wonderful recipe and cooking websites. I have a list of my cookbooks in the next section, and those can get you started in your search for recipes that fit your tastes.

- BurnFatNotSugar.com (Ted Naimen, MD)
- Cookingketowithkristie.com (Kristie Sullivan, PhD)
- DietDoctor.com (Andreas Eenfeldt, MD)
- DJFoodie.com (DJ Foodie)
- DrBerry.com (Ken Berry, MD)
- Ericwestmanmd.com (Eric Westman, MD)
- Garytaubes.com (Gary Taubes)
- HealthfulPursuit.com (Leann Vogel)
- IDMprogram.com (Jason Fung, MD)
- Ketogenic-Diet-Resource.com (Ellen Davis, MS)
- Ketogenic.com (Ryan Lowery, PhD)
- Ketonutrition.org (Dominic D'Agostino, PhD)
- Ketorevolution.org (Lisa Carroll)
- Lowcarbzen.com (Dixie Vogel)
- Obesityunderstood.com (Robert Cywes, MD)
- Packyourownbag.com (Renée Jones)
- PaleoLeap.com (Sebastien Noel)
- Racheldee.com (Rachael D. Thomas)
- TuitNutrition.com (Amy Berger, MS, CNS)
- Virtahealth.com (where you will find information about Drs. Sarah Hallberg, Stephen Phinney and Jeff Volek)

COOKBOOKS

Many of these cookbooks also have sections that explain ketogenic or low carb eating. Some contain an autobiography of the author's journey or a roadmap to the eating style. They are, however, primarily cookbooks. I also include Paleo cookbooks as they are highly helpful for finding family-friendly low carb recipes and work especially well with TRANSITIONS STEPS 1 and 2.

- Ale, K. (2020) *Keto Slow Cooker Cookbook*, PaleoHacks, LLC.

- Ballantyne, S. (2014) *The Paleo Approach Cookbook*, Las Vegas: Victory Belt Publishing, Inc.
- Barot, M. and Gaedke, M. (2018) *Keto Made Easy*, Las Vegas: Victory Belt Publishing, Inc.
- Brown, C. (2017) 101 *Keto Beverages*.
- Brown, C. (2017) *Keto for the Holidays*.
- Brown, C. (2017) *The Keto Soup Bowl*.
- Brown, C. (2017) *The Keto Crockpot*.
- Credicott, T. (2013) *Make Ahead Paleo*, Las Vegas: Victory Belt Publishing, Inc.
- Dispirito, R. (2020) *Rocco's Keto Comfort Food Diet*, New York, Rodale.
- Emmerich, M. (2017) *Keto Comfort Foods*, Las Vegas: Victory Belt Publishing, Inc.
- Fragoso, S. (2011) *Everyday Paleo*, Las Vegas: Victory Belt Publishing, Inc.
- Fragoso, S. (2012) *Everyday Paleo Family Cookbook,* Las Vegas: Victory Belt Publishing, Inc.
- Fragoso, S. (2013) *Everyday Paleo Italian Cuisine*, Las Vegas: Victory Belt Publishing, Inc.
- Gower, C. (2012) *Paleo Slow Cooking*, Las Vegas: Victory Belt Publishing, Inc.
- Holley, K. (2018) *30-Minute Ketogenic Cooking*, Las Vegas: Victory Belt Publishing, Inc.
- Holley, K. (2018) *Craveable Keto Cookbook*, Las Vegas: Victory Belt Publishing, Inc.
- Joulwan, M. (2013) *Well Fed 2, Austin*, Smudge Publishing, LLC.
- Ketchum, C. (2018) *Easy Keto Dinners,* Las Vegas: Victory Belt Publishing, Inc.
- Menegaz, V. (2016) *The Everything Big Book of Fat Bombs,* Avon: F+W Media, Inc.
- Moore, J. and Emmerich, M. (2015) *The Ketogenic Cookbook*, Las Vegas: Victory Belt Publishing, Inc.
- Sanfilippo, D. (2012) *Practical Paleo*, Las Vegas: Victory Belt Publishing, Inc.
- Santos-Prowse, R. (2017) *The Ketogenic Mediterranean Diet*, Berkeley: Ulysses Press.
- Slajerova, M. (2017) *Quick Keto, Beverly:* Quarto Publishing Group USA Inc.
- Sullivan, K. (2017) *A Journey Worth Taking*. Createspace.
- Sullivan, K. (2019) *Crazy Busy Keto*, Las Vegas: Victory Belt Publishing, Inc.
- Sullivan, K. (2018) *Keto Living Day by Day,* Las Vegas: Victory Belt Publishing, Inc.
- Sullivan, K. (2019) *Keto Gatherings,* Las Vegas: Victory Belt Publishing, Inc.
- Tam, M. and Fong, H. (2013) *Nom Nom Paleo*, Kansas City, Andres McMeel Publishing.
- Walker, D. (2013) *Against the Grain*, Las Vegas: Victory Belt Publishing, Inc.

- Walker, D. (2013) *Against the Grain, Meals Made Simple*, Las Vegas: Victory Belt Publishing, Inc.

- Weber, L. (2013) *Ultimate Keto Cookbook*, Morton Grove: Publications International, Ltd.

- Weeks, C., Boumrar, N., and Sanfilippo, D. (2014) *Mediterranean Paleo Cooking*, Las Vegas: Victory Belt Publishing, Inc.

- William, K.E. (2016) *DJ Foodie: Taking Out the Carbage*.

- William, K.E. (2017) *DJ Foodie: The Fakery*.

REFERENCES

Although citations are not specified in the body of this book, the references below support the statements and ideas made herein. Some of the books listed here contain recipes but are not primarily cookbooks. Cookbooks are listed in the Resource section.

Anton, S. et al. (2010) "Effects of stevia, aspartame, and sucrose on food intake, sensitivity, and postprandial glucose and insulin levels," *Appetite*, 55:1.

Atkins, R. (2002) *Dr. Atkins' New Diet Revolution*, New York: HarperCollins Publishers.

Aubrey, A. (2014) *"Don't Fear the Fat: Experts Question Saturated Fat Guidelines,"* NPR: The Salt – What's on Your Plate, March.

Benton, E. (2018) *Chasing Cupcakes,* Primal Potential.

Berger, A. (2017) *The Alzheimer's Antidote*, White River Junction: Chelsea Green Publishing.

Berger, A. (2020) *The Stall Slayer,* Cheyenne, Wyoming: Gutsy Badger Publishing.

Berry, K. (2019) *Lies My Doctor Told Me*, Las Vegas: Victory Belt Publishing, Inc.

Bjarnadottir, A. (2016) *"The 14 Most Common Signs of Gluten Intolerance,"* Healthline, September 29.

Bloomer, R. et al. (2016) "Blood glucose and insulin response to artificially- and sugar-sweetened sodas in healthy men," *Integrative Food, Nutrition and Metabolism*, 3:1.

Bowden, J. (2013) *Living Low Carb*, New York: Sterling.

Bowthorpe, J. (2011) *Stop the Thyroid Madness*, Laughing Grape Publishing.

Byrne C. and Targher, G. (2015) "NAFLD: a multisystem disease," *Journal of Hepatology*, 62:1(Suppl).

Campos, M. (2017) "Leaky gut: What is it and what does it mean for you?" *Harvard Health Publishing,* September 22.

Castillo, B. *The Life Coach School.* Self-Coaching Scholars.

Chowdhury, R. et al. (2014) "Association of dietary, circulating, and supplement fatty acids with coronary risk," *Annals of Internal Medicine*, 160:6.

Cole, W. (2018) *Keto•Tarian*, New York: Penguin Random House, LLC.

Connecticut College (2013) "Are Oreos addictive? Research says yes," *ScienceDaily,* 15 October.

Cummins, I. and Gerber, J. (2018) *Eat Rich Live Long*, Las Vegas: Victory Belt Publishing, Inc.

David, J. (2005) *The Slow Down Diet*, Rochester: Healing Arts Press.

Davis, E. and Runyan, K. (2017) *Conquer Type 2 Diabetes With A Ketogenic Diet*, Cheyenne, Gutsy Badger Publishing.

Davis, E. (2017) *Fight Cancer with a Ketogenic Diet, Third Edition.* Cheyenne, Gutsy Badger Publishing

Davis, E. (2017) *The Ketogenic Diet for Type 1 Diabetes* Cheyenne, Gutsy Badger Publishing

Davis, W. (2011) *Wheat Belly*, New York: Penguin Random House, LLC.

Ely A. and Cusack A. (2015) "The Binge and the Brain," *Cerebrum*, Oct 1.

Fasano, A. et al. (2015) "Nonceliac gluten sensitivity," *Gastroenterology*, 148:6.

Forleo, M. (2019) *Everything is Figureoutable*, New York: Portfolio/Penguin.

Freed, D. (1999) "Do Dietary Lectins Cause Disease?" *British Medical Journal,* 318:7190.

Fung, J. (2018) *The Diabetes Code*, Vancouver/Berkeley: Greystone Books.

Fung, J. (2016) *The Obesity Code*, Vancouver/Berkeley: Greystone Books.

Fung, J. and Moore, J. (2016) *The Complete Guide to Fasting*, Las Vegas: Victory Belt Publishing, Inc.

Gundry, S. (2008) *Dr. Gundry's Diet Revolution,* New York: Three Rivers Press.

Gunnars, K. (2020) "How many carbs should you eat per day to lose weight?" *Healthline*, April 2.

Gustin, A. and Irvin, C. (2009) *Keto Answ__ers*, Four Pillar Health.

Hansen, K. (2016) *Brain Over Binge, Recovery Guide*, Camellia Publishing, LLC.

Harcombe Z. US dietary guidelines: is saturated fat a nutrient of concern? *Br J Sports Med.* 2019 Nov;53(22):1393-1396.

Harvard Heart Letter (2011) "Abundance of fructose not good for the liver, heart," *Harvard Health Publishing*, September.

Hormone Health Network. (2020) "*Leptin | Hormone Health Network*," Hormone.org, Endocrine Society, 13 September.

Indiana University. (2010) "Sticking to diets is about more than willpower — complexity matters," *Science Daily*, January 15.

Izadi V, Saraf-Bank S, Azadbakht L. Dietary intakes and leptin concentrations. *ARYA Atherosclerosis.* 2014 Sep;10(5):266-272.

Jaruvongvanich V. et al. (2016) "Non-alcoholic fatty liver disease is associated with coronary artery calcification: A systematic review and meta-analysis," *Digest of Liver Disease*, 48:12.

Mandi, E. (2020) "What's the Difference Between Sugar and Sugar Alcohol?" *Healthline*, March 24.

Mata, J. et al. (2010) "When weight management lasts. Lower perceived rule complexity increases adherence," *Appetite*, 54:1.

May, M. (2014) *Eat What You Love, Love What You Eat*, Austin: Greenleaf Book Group Press.

May, M. and Anderson, K. (2014) *Eat What You Love, Love What You Eat for Binge Eating*, Phoenix: Am I Hungry Publishing.

May, M. and Fletcher, M. (2012) *Eat What You Love, Love What You Eat with Diabetes*, Oakland: New Harbinger Publications, Inc.

Moore, J. and Moore, C. (2019) *Real Food Keto*, Las Vegas: Victory Belt Publishing, Inc.

Moore, J. and Westman, E. (2013) *Cholesterol Clarity*, Las Vegas: Victory Belt Publishing, Inc.

Moore, J. and Westman, E. (2014) *Keto Clarity*, Las Vegas: Victory Belt Publishing, Inc.

Nally, A. and Moore, J. (2018) *The Keto Cure*, Las Vegas: Victory Belt Publishing, Inc.

National Institute of Diabetes and Digestive and Kidney Diseases. *Modification of Diet in Renal Disease (MDRD) study, 1989-1993*, National Institutes of Health.

O'Hearn, A. (2019) "*Vitamin C On The Keto Diet (Everything You Need To Know),*" Nutrita.App, July.

Page, D. D. (2019) *Positively Unstoppable*, New York: Rodale.

Perlmutter, D. (2018) *Grain Brain*, New York: Little, Brown Spark.

Petre, A. (2020) "Artificial Sweeteners: Good or Bad?" *Healthline*, August 19.

Pitman, K.R. (2013) *Overcoming Sugar Addiction*, Livingston: Five Oceans Press.

Ramsden, C. E. et al. (2016). "Re-evaluation of the traditional diet-heart hypothesis: analysis of recovered data from Minnesota Coronary Experiment (1968-73)," *British Medical Journal* (Clinical research ed.), 353:i1246.

Roth, G. (1993) *Feeding the Hungry Heart*, New York: Penguin Books.

Roth, G. (1989) *Why Weight*, New York: Penguin Books.

Schuna, C. (2018) "*How Much Protein is Too Much for a Female?*" SFGate, December 6.

Sinha, R. "*Inflammation: The Real Cause of Heart Attacks,*" Sutter Health.

Sisson, M. (2017) *The Keto Reset Diet*, New York: Harmony Books.

Spritzler, F. (2019) *Autophagy: Body's Natural Intelligence for Anti-Aging and Healing*. PG Publishing, LLC.

Spritzler, F. (2016) "*15 Easy Ways to Reduce Your Carbohydrate Intake,*" Healthline, June 13.

Stephens, G. (2107) *Delay, Don't Deny: Living an Intermittent Fasting Lifestyle,* Createspace.

Stephens, G. (2017) *Feast Without Fear: Food and the Delay, Don't Deny Lifestyle*. Createspace.

Streit, L. (2018) "*Micronutrients: Types, Functions, Benefits and More,*" Healthline, September.

Taubes, G. (2007) *Good Calories, Bad Calories*, New York: Anchor Books.

Taubes, G. (2016) *The Case Against Sugar*, Toronto: Knopf and Knopf.

Taubes, G. (2010) *Why We Get Fat and What to Do About It*, New York: Anchor Books.

Teicholz, N. (2014) *The Big Fat Surprise*, New York: Simon & Schuster.

Tribole, E. and Resch, E. (1995) *Intuitive Eating*, New York: St. Martin's Griffin.

Volek, J. and Phinney, S. (2011) T*he Art and Science of Low Carbohydrate Living*, Miami: Beyond Obesity, LLC.

Volek, J. and Phinney, S. (2012) *The Art and Science of Low Carbohydrate Performance*, Miami: Beyond Obesity, LLC.

Vogel, D. (2016) *Weight Loss Zen*, Lakeway, TX.

Vogel, L. (2019) *Keto for Women*, Las Vegas: Victory Belt Publishing, Inc.

Vogel, L. (2017) *The Keto Diet*, Las Vegas: Victory Belt Publishing, Inc.

Weigle, D. et al. (2003) "Roles of Leptin and Ghrelin in the Loss of Body Weight Caused by a Low Fat, High Carbohydrate Diet," *The Journal of Clinical Endocrinology & Metabolism*, 88: 4.

Weinberg, S. L. (2004) "The Diet-Heart Hypothesis: A Critique," *Journal of the American College of Cardiology*, 43:5.

Westman, E. and Berger, A. (2020) *"End Your Carb Confusion,"* Las Vegas: Victory Belt Publishing, Inc.

Westman, E., Phinney, S. and Volek, J. (2010) T*he New Atkins for a New You*, New York: Touchstone.

Westman, E. (2013) *A Carbohydrate Ketogenic Diet Manual*. Createspace.

Wilson, J. and Lowery, R. (2017) *The Ketogenic Bible*, Las Vegas: Victory Belt Publishing, Inc.

Winters, N. and Kelley, J.H. (2017) *The Metabolic Approach to Cancer,* White River Junction: Chelsea Green Publishing.

ABOUT THE AUTHOR

Miriam Hatoum, also known as Granny Keto, began her low carb and keto journey in the summer of 2016, when she had her lightbulb moment listening to Gary Taubes's *Why We Get Fat and What to Do About It*. Within a year her cholesterol, triglycerides, fasting insulin and blood sugar were all normal. She embarked on the path to becoming a certified health coach so that she could help other people in the most successful way possible. Her insight on what it takes to be successful – even when facing a pantry full of cookies and gummy bears – is evident in the Practical Applications and Mindfulness Practices in this book. Miriam holds M.A. and M.Ed. degrees and uses both in her three-pillar system for *Breaking Free From Diet Prison: A Common Sense Approach to Keto and Low Carb*.

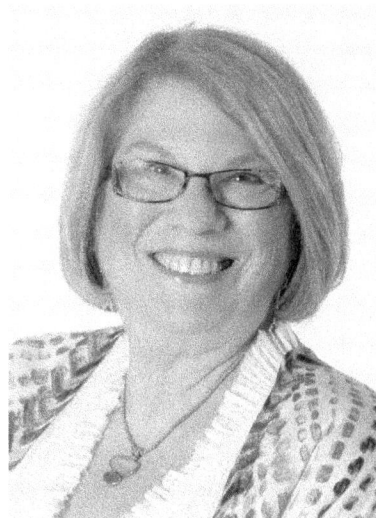

The seven-module course, *Breaking Free From Diet Prison: The Roadmap to Low Carb and Keto Success*, is available on Miriam's website at miriamhatoum.com. The course, based on this book, has hundreds of colored slides along with video narrations by the author. In-depth explanations of practical applications will make this way of eating a success for you and your family. She and her husband are former owners of Sindbad Restaurant in New York and you will find many Mediterranean-inspired recipes for keto and low carb also on her website, miriamhatoum.com. You can also find Miriam at:

- Pinterest at https://www.pinterest.com/miriam_hatoum/

- Facebook at Breaking Free From Diet Prison (https://www.facebook.com/TeamGrannyKeto)

- Facebook (Group) at Granny Keto's Transitions Team: https://www.facebook.com/groups/gktransitionsteam

- YouTube at https://www.youtube.com/channel/UCSiwv4srfT7c6PgnNkCbtUg

- Instagram: https://www.instagram.com/breakingfreefromdietprison/

www.ingramcontent.com/pod-product-compliance
Lightning Source LLC
Chambersburg PA
CBHW080418030426

42335CB00020B/2497